M

IRON LUNG

A Biography of Polio.

by Forrest Maready

Besides historical references, the names, places, and accounts mentioned in this book are used anonymously. Any resemblance to actual persons, living or dead, is entirely coincidental.

FEELS LIKE FIRE!

 Published in the United States by Feels Like Fire, an imprint of Feels Like Fire.

ISBN 978-1717583673

Printed in the United States of America

Also by Forrest Maready:

Crooked:Man-made Disease Explained, 2018
My Incredible Opinion Vol. 1, 2016
My Incredible Opinion Vol. 2, 2017
Massa Damnata, 2017

"I breathe."
– Barret Hoyt, after being placed in an iron lung.

The Iron Lung

OF THE MANY IRON LUNG PHOTOGRAPHS TO come out of the 1930s and 40s, one stands out as especially haunting. It looks to be a bedroom. In the background sits a small dresser topped with a doily, family pictures, and a perfume atomizer. A large sheet covers the right side, presumably to hide the bedding, which has been leaned against the wall to make room for what lies in the center: a gritty, cobbled together iron lung, made from spare parts one might find in any auto garage. The central component is a discarded 10 gallon drum of Veedol Motor Oil, lying on its side across two chairs. A makeshift bellows has been attached to an electric motor in an attempt to push air in and out of the cylinder. The whole affair is bolted down into an otherwise unblemished wooden floor—a subtle but stark indicator of the desperation involved in this scene.

There are many pictures throughout American history of men enjoying the results of their clever time-saving, work-reducing inventions. This picture is different. A man—likely the inventor—sits beside the contraption, his hands covered in grease, looking tenderly at the person inhabiting the barrel. He is presumably a new father and is desperately trying to save his child's life. Inside the Veedol barrel lies an infant, its tiny head —barely half the size of his grease-covered hand—the only part of its body that is visible.

Whether this child was suffering from polio, or simply the effects of a premature birth, we can only guess. Whatever it was, in the 1900s people—particularly children—were being stricken down with paralysis, and mothers, fathers, doctors, and nurses were doing anything they could to save them. In the past, a sick child could be held, rocked, or given powders or syrup recommended by the doctor. In the paralytic polio era, none of these seemed to work—there was nothing one could do besides sit and wait.

During the peak of the polio epidemic in the 1950s, there were 1,157 iron lungs in operation in the United States. Although their use was limited, the psychological impact they have had on the public's perception of polio has been immense. These gargantuan iron coffins which made the humans inside—with the exception of their head—invisible have shaped our knowledge about this mysterious disease like nothing else. Most people have heard of polio and have some idea what its symptoms are. Many people have seen pictures of otherwise healthy looking children, their legs and feet bound up in casts and splints to help them walk. But nearly everyone has burned into their mind a few black and white images of disembodied humans, floating inside iron sarcophaguses as if they were part of some giant magic show—their bodies waiting to be cut in half and put back together again.

For many inside the iron lungs, the paralysis would disappear after several weeks or months, and they might return to some semblance of a normal life. But for the rest of humanity, the images of victims stuck inside the iron lung would forever change the way they thought about disease and medicine.

* * *

There is another story about polio that is not often told. The black and white images of people in iron lungs are often as far as many people's recollections will take them. It was a terrible disease with a terrible diagnosis and an even more terrible treatment. Many books have been written about it—specifically, the fear and panic that overtook much of the world in the mid 1900s and the scientists who completed their heroic quest for a vaccine. It's a tale that any human would enjoy hearing—the conquest of a dreaded disease by the unrelenting perseverance and cunning of our best and brightest minds. David Oshinsky's *Polio, An American Story,* won the 2006 Pulitzer Prize for history. Many other books on the subject are similarly appreciated. The polio vaccine sits at the top of many lists ranking the greatest medical achievements in human history and the decades-long account of its creation makes for riveting drama.

But lost amidst the jubilation of Salk's injected polio vaccine in 1955 and Sabin's oral vaccine in 1961 is an intriguing riddle—a question whose answer is fascinating to those who are deeply curious about polio: What happened before the vaccine? What caused a previously innocuous virus to begin paralyzing people—seemingly randomly at first in the early 1800s, then more frequently in epidemic form in the late 1800s and early 1900s? For all the fanfare of victory over the dreaded disease, few seem interested in finding out why the vaccine was necessary at all.

Besides a few isolated cases of paralysis that appear sporadically within the medical literature, polio was completely unknown to most physicians—so rare, in fact, that doctors of New York City in 1916 would need to attend classes to learn how to recognize its symptoms, as most of them had never seen a single case themselves. In 1932, an international group trying to make sense of polio's rise confessed, "No circumstance in the history of poliomyelitis is so baffling as its change, during the last two decades of the nineteenth century, from a sporadic to an epidemic disease."[1]

The increasingly large outbreaks of the illness were not the only concern. The selective nature of those it targeted baffled those who studied it. In 1943, years before he would perfect the oral polio vaccine, a perplexed Albert Sabin wrote a colleague from the Philippines:

> *"The only mystery as I see it, is why the incidence is so much higher among [our] troops than among the natives."*[2]

Sabin had temporarily halted his polio work and joined the U.S. Army in conducting infectious disease research abroad during the second World War. The paralysis that had gripped young children every summer in the United States (and a few other first world countries) seemed remarkably absent elsewhere—more confusing because local Filipinos tested positive for poliovirus while their incidence of *paralysis* was nearly zero. It was a pattern that vexes researchers to this day—where disease and death often tracked the abysmal sanitation and nutrition of the poor, polio seemed to affect the rich and well-to-do. The better the sanitation, the more frequently paralysis would occur.

* * *

Polio is, in a morbid way, a disease of the dead—a living person cannot be conclusively diagnosed with polio. A clinical diagnosis can be made based on the patient's symptoms. A spinal tap can be performed to check for elevated spinal fluid pressure or white blood cell counts. Sophisticated antibody tests can be conducted to deduce a recent poliovirus infection. But to conclusively diagnose someone with polio, you must obtain a cross-section of their spinal column and place it under a microscope—a procedure seldom performed on the living. After peering around, deep within the neurons, you may find what you are looking for—grey lesions of decaying nervous tissue. If you are able to find these lesions, you must then take a much closer look—possibly with an electron microscope—and make a determination if they were caused by inflammation from the poliovirus.

The body is very good at protecting its central nervous system from invaders. For these lesions of polio to have occurred, a virus had to have gotten past several layers of defense from the immune system—through the mucosal tissue in the intestines, into the blood, and possibly beyond the blood brain barrier, finding purchase in the bottom of the spinal cord, as was its common point of entry.

Throughout human history, the body appeared suitably equipped to handle poliovirus infections—its presence was more likely to create immunity than paralysis or any other problem. Something changed, starting in the late 1800s, which turned this once harmless infection into a frequent killer. The story of what caused this formerly trivial virus to transform into a monster is as important as what seemed to tame it.

The story of polio *before* the vaccine may be the most important part specifically because of the nature of what may have created the problem in the first place. Humans tend towards hubris rather than humility, a trait that has likely created as much suffering as any bacteria or virus. While the valiant story of man over microbe is undoubtedly compelling, an honest look into the nooks and crannies of what caused the epidemics of polio is deeply humbling. Man at his best can inspire like no other. Man at his worst, can destroy. Man in his natural state—with seemingly more reluctance to look himself in the mirror and admit his mistakes, the more noble his intent that caused them—that condition may be most crippling of them all.

the MOTH in the IRON LUNG

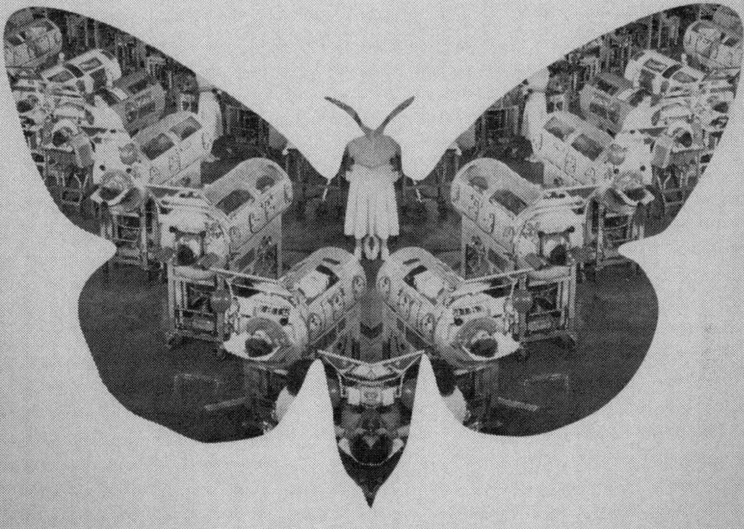

Forrest Maready

Author of **Crooked:Man-Made Disease Explained**

Chapter One

Boston, 1869

It was spring 1869. Like many other cities around the country, Boston, Massachusetts was still recovering from the devastation of the Civil War. Though the conflict had ended four years earlier, a huge musical celebration called the *National Peace Jubilee* would soon take place in a newly built coliseum covering over four and a half acres—the largest structure in all 37 states of the country.

The event would last five days and was described in its official program as "The Grandest Musical Festival Ever Known In The History Of The World." It would feature an enormous pipe organ, a 525-member orchestra, a wind band with 486 performers, and 100 different choral groups totaling nearly

11,000 singers. Over 50,000 men, women, and children would fill the stands each day—not only to benefit the widows and orphans of the war, but to "Commemorate the Restoration of Peace Throughout the Land."

Red, white, and blue bunting hung throughout the massive wooden structure. A huge bass drum, eight feet in diameter, featured hand-painted lettering that proclaimed, "LET US HAVE PEACE." Other smaller drums displayed the less inspirational message of "GILMORE," the name of the event's conductor and organizer, Patrick Gilmore—better known for his rousing Civil War tune, "When Johnny Comes Marching Home."

After an opening prayer and a 45-minute address on restoration and peace, the pipe organ—powered by a gas engine outside—unleashed a din of air and sound into the room as the familiar refrains of "A Mighty Fortress is Our God" brought everyone to their feet. A soldier from the war, Oliver Wendell Holmes, penned the words to a three-stanza "Hymn of Peace" commissioned for the occasion:

Angel of peace, thou hast wandered too long;
Spread thy white wings to the sunshine of love!
Come while our voices are blended in song,
Fly to our ark like the storm-beaten dove—
Fly to our ark on the wings of the dove;
Speed o'er the far-sounding billows of song,
Crowned with the olive leaf garland of love;
Angel of peace, thou hast waited too long!

Singing had been taught in New England schools as

earnestly as reading or arithmetic, so when the first half of the concert concluded with "The Star-Spangled Banner," the opening stanza began with the unfathomable rumble of twenty-five hundred basses singing in unison. By the end of the third stanza, all the singers and performers had joined in, even a cannon outside the hall, firing in time—an effect for which United States president Ulysses Grant proclaimed his "favorite part of the music." Men stood and clapped, women shook their handkerchiefs in the air, and children begged their parents for more.

It was the grandest musical experience the world had ever seen. Newspapers around the country—many who had ridiculed the ostentatious promise of cannon fire and anvil-playing firefighters—were forced to admit the overall effect of the five-day affair was nothing but a resounding success. Patrick Gilmore's Jubilee had perfectly encapsulated the joy and elation everyone felt as the country emerged from four years of brutal fighting still united. The war was officially over, and all of Boston and the other great cities across the land were eager to embrace the seemingly infinite promise of a unified country.

* * *

Although the nation would not sacrifice so many in military conflict for many years, a new menace was emerging, just six miles away from Gilmore's grand coliseum—a scourge that would claim the lives or health of millions around the world for the next century. While the Civil War had targeted mostly young men with death, this threat was different—it would often mark children as its prey and though many would die, those that didn't were frequently left lame or crippled for the rest of their lives.

Just north of the National Peace Jubilee, across Boston's Charles and Mystic Rivers, a man was fumbling through the grass and bushes that lined the side of his small two-story house. Neighbors walked by and remarked at his frantic search as he clawed through blades of grass on his hands and knees. It was a pleasant spring day, but the wind had picked up, frustrating his efforts.

Clearly distraught, he went back to the window from where his search had begun. Just a few minutes earlier, he had placed a mass of moth eggs on the kitchen sill when a gust of wind lifted them up in the air and out into the yard. He burst through the front door and leapt off the porch in an attempt to collect them before the mass broke apart, littering the yard with hundreds of tiny eggs.

It was too late. He groped through foliage looking for signs of the furry brown sac, but it was gone. The eggs contained inside had probably separated and been carried up into the wind. They could have landed anywhere in his yard—or his neighbors. He had lost other eggs, caterpillars, and moths before, but they were native species—perfectly suited for the local environment due to thousands of years of natural selection. These were not. He knew enough about moths and their voracious appetite to be severely distressed. The fact that these were an invasive species of moth—brought to the United States from Europe—made it all the more troubling.

He brushed the dirt and grass from his knees, returned inside and sat down at the kitchen table. The Civil War was over and cotton had returned to the North. The soaring demand for silk had evaporated and years of his painstaking silkworm research would count for nothing. He checked his sleeves and noticed a single egg, one of probably five-hundred, nestled within the folds of his cuffs. It was time to move, he thought—closer to the city. He didn't need acres of forest in which to run his experiments any longer.

* * *

A few summers later, a new family had moved into his house and several curious creatures appeared on the clapboard siding. To the children playing outside, they would have appeared to be just another caterpillar. But with their hairy bodies and twin sets of blue and red dots along their back, they were anything but. They were *Lymantria dispar dispar*, the larval form of the gypsy moth—an insect that had been causing devastation in Europe for years. The man who had let them escape knew the ruin they might cause to the surrounding area if they weren't destroyed. However, neither he or the new family living at 27 Myrtle Street, could have imagined the furry caterpillar crawling along the side their house would inadvertently set the stage for epidemics of the most famous disease in modern history—polio.

37 years earlier…

Chapter Two

England, 1832

It was 1832 and the age of wonder was overtaking much of Europe. Humphry Davy had isolated potassium, sodium, and created artificial light that could be safely taken into coal mines filled with gas. His colleague, Michael Faraday, had just discovered electromagnetic induction, a concept which would become the driving force within electric motors and generators.

Across St. George's Channel, an Irish physician designed a device that would allow for artificial respiration. It was a large wooden box in which the patient could sit upright, their head and neck protruding through an airtight opening on the top. A bellows was attached to a slowly reciprocating piston and its movement would temporarily create a vacuum inside the box, forcing the patient's chest to expand and draw in air through their mouth. As the piston traveled to the other end of its throw, it would squeeze the bellows, compressing air into the box—forcing the patient to exhale. Two small windows allowed the operator to look inside and observe the effects of the mechanism.

Although he did not understand the idiosyncrasies of oxygen exchange within the lungs, it was assumed this method of artificial respiration might be enough to keep someone alive who could not breathe on their own. Future designs would allow the patient to lie down flat on their back rather than sit on a small stool within the box—a marked improvement no doubt —but the general concept of assisted breathing would remain unchanged for many years.

The reason the Irish physician developed this device was for a common problem the fishermen who braved the North Sea and Atlantic oceans often faced—drowning. Mouth to mouth, or *rescue breathing,* was well known and practiced, in addition to crude instruments like a handheld bellows, but both presented problems. Physicians of the day thought most oxygen was removed from the air by the lungs and consequently believed the recycled air of rescue breathing was insufficient to sustain life. The bellows technique provided little feedback to the operator and could easily rupture the lungs if too much pressure was applied, particularly with children.

Because of this, a more natural way of simulating the breathing process was sought, and the physician's design would be replicated and improved upon many times over the next hundred years. Back in England, Davy and Faraday's discoveries would both later contribute to artificial respiration

—Davy's, in the form of increased coal mining and the asphyxiation that often accompanied this type of work, and Faraday, in the form of electric motors that would power future iterations of the wooden breathing box called *iron lungs*.

While drownings had been a constant threat since man had taken to water, and Europe's recent drive deep underground in the search for coal would create a new manner of suffocation, the disease which artificial respiration machines would become synonymous with was all but unheard of in 1832. Just three years later, that would begin to change.

* * *

In the center of England in a small town called Worksop, a physician named Charles Badham felt compelled to write about a disturbing illness he had witnessed during the summer of 1835. Four children, all under the age of three, had come down with paralysis, mainly in their legs, or "lower extremities." All of them appeared healthy with the exception of "an unusual appearance of the eyes, which... appeared to be turned inwards."[3]

Badham documented the particular symptoms of these children because it was something he had never heard of. Apparently his father, also a physician, wasn't familiar with it either. Paralysis was not out of the ordinary at the time, but the fact it had struck four different people—all of them under the age of three—felt to him, remarkable. That their health was otherwise unimpaired was also odd. Although he asked other doctors to get in touch and offer him advice on how to treat this new phenomenon, he would get few responses.

A physician in Germany read Badham's account and began to notice similar symptoms amongst patients he and his colleagues were treating. By 1840, he had accumulated fourteen different accounts of people—mostly children—who had experienced paralysis of their legs, sometimes arms. Like Badham, he was struck by their youth and otherwise robust health. He created a 78-page monograph, complete with illustrations of the stricken children, in an attempt to draw attention to this strange disorder which had apparently gone unnoticed until recently.

* * *

Sporadic reports of *infantile paralysis* would dot the medical literature for the next fifty years. A child here, an infant there. Always during the summer, almost always the young and healthy. Patterns of the disease began to appear—paralysis, usually in the legs, sometimes the arms. Usually boys, though not always. Mobility was sometimes fully regained, sometimes partially. Other symptoms commonly surfaced alongside the new illness that defied explanation. Teething was almost always mentioned as either a cause or contributing factor, as was overheating or over-exertion.

Thankfully, whatever the illness was, it was completely rare. Rare—at least—until the summer of 1894, when just north of Boston in a small New England town in Vermont, polio would strike with a vengeance that no one had ever seen before.

Chapter Three

Boston, 1856

THE YEAR WAS 1856. GETTING ACROSS THE Atlantic Ocean was not an easy task, even for those with money. For most, they would make the trip on packet ships—small ocean liners whose principal cargo was parcels of mail. Humans often rode along below deck in steerage—a large common room with tiny wooden bunks around the periphery in which to sleep.

Etienne Trouvelot and his wife anxiously boarded one of these ships. They were leaving France for the promise of America, a few of their precious possessions crammed into the steamer trunk left with the porter at the foot of the gangplank. Unaware bedding was not provided, Trouvelot had to buy them from vendors running alongside the vessel, purchasing a cheaper wood shaving mattress for himself and an upgrade for his pregnant wife—a mattress filled with seaweed and a tiny pillow sewn into one end. Other vendors sold coffee tins, silverware and any other knick-knacks which might be useful on the ten-day passage across the mercurial Atlantic ocean.

In front of them, nervous parents and their children were hustled down the nearly vertical ladders below deck where they would spend much of the next few days of their life. These were not huge vessels with massive drafts that could dampen a large storm—they were small, 200- to 300-foot steam-powered ocean liners. Except for the seasoned crew, all on board would brace and steady themselves for every wave they crested. As Trouvelot and his wife made their way across the darkened room and looked for the bunk in which they would sleep, wind peeled off the water and through the portholes along the side of the ship, wafting foul odors from below—a harbinger of but one of the many hardships that lay ahead.

In steerage, daily food allotments were provided, but cooking was left to the passengers—hungry families fighting with each other over access to the stoves and boiling water. A guide from a British ship around that time provides a glimpse into what their allocations might have been:

> *"The following quantities at least of water and provisions to be issued daily will be supplied by the master of the ship, as required by law, viz.: To each statute adult 3 quarts of water daily, exclusive of what is necessary for cooking those articles required by the Passengers' Act to be issued in a cooked state, and a weekly allowance of provisions according to the following scale-3% pounds of bread, 1% pounds of fresh bread, 1 pound of flour, 1% pounds*

oatmeal, 1% pounds rice, 3 pounds potatoes, 1% pounds peas, 4 ounces raisins, 2 pounds beef, 1% pounds pork, 1 pound fish, 2 ounces tea, 2 ounces coffee or cocoa, 1 pound sugar, 1 gill molasses, 1 gill vinegar, 3 ounces salt, 1 ounce mustard and pepper.—Children under 8 receive one-half the above."

Dining was a decidedly pedestrian affair. There were no tablecloths or wooden chairs, but instead long tables tied to the ceiling which were lowered into the center of the room during mealtimes. Wooden planks were affixed to iron posts on either side for seating. As the journey progressed, more empty seats appeared every day—passengers learned they could bribe the porters above for access to some of the meals prepared for the crew. Everything was for sale, illicitly or otherwise—even clean water for washing plates and silverware had a price some were willing to pay.

To pass the time, passengers would dance, sing, and share books or magazines. A rowdy group of girls held high-kicking contests deep into the night, marking their efforts in chalk on the wall. Others would share personal stories of hope—where they had come from, or visions of the better lives they hoped to lead in the promised land across the sea. It is not known what drove Trouvelot to America, but his choice of Boston was probably no accident—it was the center of scientific research in the new country, and its crown jewel, Harvard College, had an impressive astronomical observatory—something in which Trouvelot was keenly interested.

On their final day of sailing, the Atlantic ocean gave them a parting gift—a raucous Nor'easter with heavy winds, rain, and slogging waves. Portholes were shut and the air quickly turned fetid. Soup and coffee kettles rattled against each other as the ship tossed to and fro. Potatoes and apples rolled across the floor. Ropes were strung across the room onto which petrified passengers could cling. Sleep was difficult in the cramped, dank conditions even without foul weather, but within the storm, it was impossible. One by one, seasickness claimed everyone.

As they pulled into the harbor, many of those on the ship stayed up through the night, eager to catch their first glimpse of America through a crowded porthole or up on deck for those who could sneak past the porters. As daylight broke, men and women were separated, lined up, and inspected for their "beauty marks," or smallpox vaccination scars. Those who didn't demonstrate a clear mark were inoculated on the spot. All were given vaccination tickets to show the health officer before they were allowed off the ship.

The gangplanks were lowered and the French immigrants peered out onto the grand view that was the Boston Harbor. The water was full of three-masted clippers, their giant sails furled safely away from the wind as black puffs of smoke began to pour out of factories that dotted the cityscape. The country was exploding and to the European newcomers, its incredible industry seemed to have unlimited resources and opportunities.

Trouvelot and his wife made their way down, anxious to retrieve their steamer trunk from the longshoremen already unloading below. They would settle in a small house just a couple of miles north of Boston in Medford, Massachusetts. It was a modest two-story, two-bedroom affair, but had a special element Trouvelot was undoubtedly excited about—acres of woodland in which he could breed and study silkworms.

Chapter Four

Boston, 1865

TROUVELOT'S SKILLS AS AN ARTIST AND LITHOGRAPHER served him well, and he was able to effect a strong reputation amongst those working within Harvard's scientific realm. Many of them spoke French, and his native command of the language only bolstered his standing. Eventually, he began to assist—gathering specimens for their growing collection of insects and composing essays on the mysterious nature of what he had amassed.

His fascination with breeding silkworms could not have come at a better time. Although most in the North would be shielded from the direct violence of the Civil War, they would become keenly aware of the scarcity of a commodity they had previously taken for granted—cotton. Without the daily imports of bales of the white fiber from the Southern states, the North was forced to look for another source of fabric.

Silk is an ancient discovery thousands of years old which requires the assistance of one of nature's glorious wonders—the metamorphosis of caterpillars. In order to transform into moths, caterpillars will spin a cocoon of one continuous strand of natural fiber a thousand yards long. After their miraculous transformation, the caterpillar will emerge from the cocoon as a moth. If you were to boil it before the moth emerges, you might unwind the loosened cocoon and combine it with others to form a thread of luxuriously soft, shiny silk. This could then be woven into ties, shirts, kimonos, and a thousand other garments.

There are very few moth varieties that create cocoons which can be used in this way—the silk is either too fragile to be unwrapped easily, or the cocoon construction is done in such a way to prevent its use. Thousands of years of silkworm domestication created a fragile, disease-prone creature that essentially depended on its captors for survival, so Trouvelot began to look for ways he might strengthen their stock by cross-breeding with other varieties.

Boston was at the center of silk trade in the United States and Trouvelot was determined to put his inquisitiveness, his location, and property to good use. The area behind his house had become a massive breeding ground for silkworms—nearly a million, according to Trouvelot. Over five acres of woodland were carefully enclosed in mesh—the netting held aloft inside by taller trees in order that one could navigate around inside unimpaired. As a result, he received frequent visitors from scientists in Boston, eager to see the efforts of his work.

Although entomologists of the day were just beginning to realize the threat that invasive species posed to native habitats, the netting was not designed to retain the silkworms as much as it was to keep predators away. Birds—particularly robins—would work their way through gaps in the netting and feast on the smooth-skinned *T. polyphemus* caterpillars within. They were a constant source of frustration, and much of Trouvelot's spare time was spent scouring the vast perimeter of netting, mending and replacing the mesh wherever the birds had found a gap.

By 1866, the Civil War had ended, but such was his progress in the understanding of silkworm crossbreeding, Trouvelot made the arduous journey back to France in order to research possible candidates for additional experiments. One of the specific traits he was looking for was a preference for oak leaves. Earlier in the 1800s, the area had been aggressively cut for lumber, and the hardy oak tree had replaced much of what was lost. Caterpillars could be extremely finicky, and if there was one thing New England had a surplus of, it was oak.

Whether by mistake or design, Trouvelot returned to Boston and later received a package of several different varieties of moth eggs. Hidden amongst them was a small, light brown egg mass that would contain a creature he had never seen before—*Lymantria dispar dispar*—a particularly devastating insect otherwise known as the gypsy moth.

Chapter Five

Philadelphia, 1867

It was 1867 in Philadelphia, and a surgeon named Charles Taylor published a short 119-page work illuminating a phenomenon that he and his colleagues had begun to notice more of: *infantile paralysis.* He was concerned not only about the age of the victims, but the rise in the number of cases.

> *"There seems to be no doubt that this disease is much more frequent now, and in this country, than formerly, and is rapidly increasing."*[4]

Like many physicians of the day, Taylor believed the increase in nervous disorders like infantile paralysis was due to exhaustion caused by the "over-activity" of the brain. Similarly, he was struck by the fact that although diseases like tuberculosis were common amongst the poor, this form of paralysis was nearly absent.

Taylor spent most of the book addressing treatments and remedies for the deformities caused by this new illness. As his comprehension of the disease was understandably deficient, he attributed the withering limbs of paralysis to a lack of blood flow. Doctors didn't realize muscles which had no active stimulation would atrophy and shrink. Additionally, the destruction of neurons which prevented muscle activity also affected the growth pattern of the bones to which they were attached, causing the wild skeletal deformities that gave rise to decades of barbaric bracing and splinting.

A puzzling cause was mentioned several times throughout the book—something that had been noted elsewhere. Both parents and doctors alike attributed the onset of paralysis to the same thing:

> *"Case 6.—T. T., aged two years and a half, was paralyzed while teething."*

Taylor made it clear at the beginning of the book that the "majority of those cases, however, have about this history: the child is getting its first molar teeth." Within the book, a father gave a personal testimony of what had happened to his daughter:

> *"My daughter Josie, who was placed under your care in May and November, 1865, and has at home followed your directions in*

wearing more or less apparatus adjusted to her partially paralyzed leg, first manifested to us that her leg was debilitated when about eighteen months of age. She walked when about a year old, then gave up walking. We attributed the fact to debility from teething. When she resumed walking, at about eighteen months of age, the weakness in one leg was discovered."[5]

Even an obscure article regarding paralysis amongst a group of children in Louisiana in 1841—thought of as possibly the first reference to polio in the United States—was called "Paralysis in Teething Children." The association with dentition was so common that many parents, having never heard the term infantile paralysis, referred to what had happened to their children as *teething paralysis*. This period in a child's life was thought of as so dangerous, some considered calling dentition itself a disease.

While the initial years of a baby's life in the 1800s were challenging, perhaps there was a legitimate reason paralysis was so often associated with teething. A popular pamphlet targeting new mothers gives a clear indication of what might have been happening:

"The period of dentition is the longest, the most difficult, and the most critical operation through which a child must pass. . . . Teething may be accompanied by various rather alarming developments, such as child-crowing, convulsions, etc., which are discussed under these headings. The general health of the child requires particular attention if these troubles are to be avoided. The bowels must be kept regular."[6]

Medical practices during that period were decidedly poor.

Popular treatments involved bleeding, leeches, noxious powders, and blistering with hot irons—all of which might be employed on infants. Regardless, nothing was administered with the zeal as was mercurial medicine and arsenical solutions. Purging—or opening up—the bowels was thought to be the proper remedy for nearly any ailment of the time. This was done aggressively with purgatives such as calomel, a mercury-containing remedy.

It is difficult for a modern human to understand the ubiquity of mercury, the earth's most toxic substance (besides plutonium), in the every day life of someone living two hundred years ago. Examine any medical literature of the 1800s and early 1900s and one will not have to look far before seeing mercury-based treatments and medicines: Mercury cyanide, mercuric iodide, mercury benzoate, and mercuric chloride. These were not concoctions sold on the back pages of newspapers by traveling salesmen who would clear town as soon as they had your money—these were commercial products produced in laboratories by large companies like Sharpe & Domme and Eli Lilly.

As medicine, mercury was as ubiquitous as aspirin is today. For example, one may think of an occasional case of conjunctivitis, or "Pink Eye," as rare, but a hundred years ago it was as frequent a problem as the common cold. Because newborn babies tended to rub their faces, poor sanitation meant a constant flow of bacteria into their eyes. As a result, mercury cyanide was a recommended treatment for conjunctivitis and continued to be used until the 1950s.

In the early 1800s, a popular medicine stormed onto the market: Steedman's Teething Powders. Each package contained eight folded up pieces of paper on which the following was written:

> *"Dose. From one to three months, the third of a powder; from three to six months, half a powder; and above that age, one powder only, and no more; for further particulars read the large bill of directions."*

Each paper contained around 47 milligrams of mercury chloride powder to be placed on the back of the infant's tongue and washed down with milk or water. While they knew the mercury could have toxic effects, the drive to clear the infant's bowels was believed so essential to their health it was thought worth the risk. As such, mercurial medicines were dispensed to infants for nearly any complaint, including the privation of teething.

Paralysis is now a known side effect of mercury poisoning, but, at the time, they would not have believed the powder to have this effect. It could also cause excessive thirst, a phenomenon noted in early accounts of polio. An excerpt from one of Charles Badham's cases in 1835 England said much:

> *The child had enjoyed uninterrupted health to the evening of her attack, with the exception (if, indeed it can be so called) of slightly augmented thirst and some drowsiness, now remembered by the mother to have preceded the seizure by two days. On the evening of the 13th the child was put to bed, having run about and amused herself as usual during the day. On the following morning her mother's attention was first attracted, in dressing her, to an unusual appearance of the eyes, which as she said, appeared to be turned inwards. A new cause of apprehension presented itself in*

> *putting the child on her feet, when it was found she could not stand. Medical advice being immediately sought for, it was thought sufficient, I understand, to keep the bowels open..."*[7]

The child's "augmented thirst" may seem inconsequential, but taken in the context of a teething child likely being administered enough mercury to poison a full-grown man, it becomes an ominous note. The inward turned eye—or *strabismus*—the mother mentioned could also be attributed to this same cause. The second of Badham's four 1835 cases also presented some troubling symptoms:

> *"Thirst, remarked also in the former case, was a more prominent symptom in this... The pupil of the left eye was dilated... This case was chiefly treated with strychnine externally applied, but without any benefit; nor did... mercurials meet with better success... The limb remains perfectly palsied and useless, though sensation has been somewhat restored."*[8]

In addition to severe thirst, the second child had one eye that was dilated and extreme fatigue—both additional signs of mercury poisoning. Lastly, the final note about her sensation being restored would indicate she had lost it, an effect which—like dilated pupils and tiredness—polio is not known for. In all four cases, the children's paralysis and other issues were treated with additional mercuric medicine amongst other objectionable prescriptions. The restoration of their health under such an assault would be miraculous.

Even Michael Underwood's description of "Debility of the Lower Extremities" in 1796—considered to be the first modern description of polio—attributes the onset of the disease to "the instance of teething or of foul bowels,"[9] a pair of events that would have no doubt been treated with mercury-based purgatives. Was the suffering of these children, labeled by modern historians as polio, actually the result of a dangerous medical practice—mercury poisoning, in the form of teething powder or other purgatives? It is impossible to say, but as the 19th century wore on and more cases of polio began to appear, additional clues emerged that would only serve to complicate the answer.

Chapter Six

Poliomyelitis

AWARENESS OF *INFANTILE PARALYSIS* CONTINUED TO GROW in Europe and the United States. Although it had not yet reached critical mass, a few physicians had become sufficiently curious with the nature of the disease that they began post-mortem examinations of those whom it had presumably killed in hopes of finding its cause. To the naked eye, an abnormality within the spinal cord was sometimes visible. With the aid of a microscope, it was unmistakable: Lesions within the spinal cord—malformed tissue preventing the nerves from working properly.

The neurons within the spinal cord are divided into two different categories—*grey matter* that runs within the center of the column, and the *white matter* that surrounds it. The lesions in children who had died from infantile paralysis were nearly always in the grey matter—the inner section of the spinal cord. For this reason, some began to call what they suspected to be the cause of infantile paralysis *poliomyelitis*. Myelitis means inflammation of the spinal cord, and polio means grey.

Poliomyelitis—or inflammation of the grey matter of the spinal cord—was a term used to describe anyone, usually infants, who had developed paralysis with no apparent cause. They didn't know why it had happened, of course, but it was a term that began to be used in medical literature to comment on what might be the source of affliction.

If a doctor was summoned to the house of a child who had woken up one morning, unable to move, the physician might tell the parents he suspected "a poliomyelitis" was involved—inflammation of the grey matter of the spinal cord. The term was employed just like we might use the terms *laceration* or *concussion*. Today, when we use the word polio (a shortened version of poliomyelitis), we are referring to a disease—paralysis caused by a specific virus called poliovirus—that came to be associated with inflammation of the spinal cord. A hundred years ago, poliomyelitis (they did not use the shortened "polio" moniker) would have been freely suggested as a cause whenever someone exhibited paralysis.

This difference may seem trivial, but it is important to understand the nomenclature from which *polio* descends because, as we will soon see, many things could elicit a poliomyelitis—not just the poliovirus.

As accounts of children stricken with poliomyelitis began to grow, another characteristic became clear—it normally affected only the front half of the grey matter of the spinal cord, a discovery confirmed under the microscope. The back half of the grey matter is responsible for conveying sensory information and children didn't typically indicate pain or sensitivity—just paralysis.

The front half of the grey matter of the spinal cord, called the *anterior horn*, communicates motor commands to the muscles—this is the area in which lesions so often appeared.[i] If the injury was constrained to the front half of the spinal cord, paralysis might occur, but without any loss of feeling. This was a significant development. In the past, paralysis, usually due to physical trauma, would typically disrupt the neurons across the front and back of the spinal cord and any loss of movement would likely have been accompanied by a corresponding loss of touch. This new phenomenon might cause complete paralysis without any loss of sensation in the affected body part.

Though a comprehensive mapping of the human body was incomplete, it was thorough enough to evoke confusion: What mechanism would cause lesions in only the front half of the spinal cord? There seemed to be no anatomical feature that might explain it. While this trait of poliomyelitis—which physicians squabbled over—may have seemed inconsequential to the parents of those children affected, another anatomical quirk emerged which would concern everyone involved even more.

i. Because of this, poliomyelitis—with no impact on sensory nerves—was sometimes referred to as "acute poliomyelitis of the anterior horn."

Chapter Seven

Boston, 1869

THE WAR HAD BEEN OVER FOR NEARLY four years, and the refrains of Patrick Gilmore's Grand Music Festival rung throughout Boston. Perhaps Trouvelot and his family were able to take the six-mile train ride into town and attend. Regardless, the tireless efforts of fence-mending and cross-breeding had begun to wear on him. Cotton was flowing freely into New England again and of all the different varieties of moth eggs he had been sent from Europe, none of them showed much promise.

Trouvelot carefully tended a stock of one particular variety—what by then he would probably have recognized as the menace from Europe—the gypsy moth. Compared to the millions of *T. polyphemus* growing behind his house, it was a tiny collection, small enough to fit under the carefully wrapped netting on a single bush. The silk from their cocoon was nearly unusable, but their ability to tolerate harsh living conditions—alongside their fondness for the oak trees so plentiful in the area—convinced Trouvelot a cross with the silkworm might be universally beneficial.

For reasons unknown, Trouvelot brought the mass containing hundreds of gypsy moth eggs inside his house and placed it on the sill of an open kitchen window. Perhaps he was preparing to ship them to another researcher, but, regardless, he would not have been purposefully careless with them—he was well aware of their voracious appetite and the damage they had been causing parts of Europe, particularly Germany. When a gust of wind blew the egg mass out into his yard, he would have instantly understood the monumental importance in him retrieving it.

The recent regrowth of millions of oak trees would provide enough tinder for the gypsy moth to spread like fire throughout New England. Even more concerning, something Trouvelot would likely not have noticed with his small stock of gypsy moths, the birds—particularly the robins—would not eat them. They were not smooth like other caterpillars. Their furry bodies were uniquely distasteful, and most of the natural predators that kept other *Lepidoptera* in check would not be able to help. Trouvelot's distress was well-placed—the gypsy moth would make for a much more formidable foe than anyone could have imagined.

Entomologists in the area began to hear word that a mass of gypsy moth eggs had escaped from Trouvelot's house. He sent letters to authorities in an attempt to warn them of the destruction they could cause. The scientific community—growing more aware of the danger of non-native species every day—sounded an alarm, but the calls for action fell on deaf ears.

The government had very little authority in the way of insects, and those who might have heard his alarm were unconvinced a seemingly innocuous silkworm would be able to cause as much harm as entomologists intimated. Whatever the case, Trouvelot's attempt to stop the spread of the gypsy moth from 27 Myrtle Street in Medford, Massachusetts, would fail.

Chapter Eight

Legs & Lungs

IF ONE WERE TO LOOK THROUGH THE isolated accounts of infantile paralysis in the 1800s, a familiar pattern will appear again and again: A precocious child, running wild one day, seemingly in perfect health, is reluctantly put to bed. During the night, the child might wake up, inconsolably thirsty. After copious amounts of water, the child eventually goes to sleep. Early in the morning, the parents are woken by the gale of a screaming child and rush to her room. She has woken from a deep sleep and is on the floor, pulling herself towards the door, unable to move her legs.

Towards the end of the 19th century, this horror story would become more commonplace. Perfectly healthy children

—stricken down during the dead of night—awoken to a terrible affliction that might hound them for the rest of their lives. While the age of those who were affected was slowly changing, the location of the paralysis was not—it was almost always their legs. Occasionally, the arms might be affected—more often the trunk or abdomen—but with most children, the worst of the paralysis was usually their lower limbs.

Why this particular section of the spinal cord would so often be targeted still baffles physicians to this day. There appears to be nothing unique, anatomically speaking, about this part of the body. It is served by the same circulatory and lymphatic vessels as the rest of the central nervous system. As the neuron fires, it is farther away from the brain than any other part of the spinal column. Even as the pathology of poliomyelitis began to become clear, new discoveries only made the puzzle more perplexing.

Regardless, in a time where hard, physical labor was the norm, the loss of one's legs would have been devastating. There were few wheelchairs available and even fewer paved roads on which their hard, wooden wheels could easily traverse. Besides the logistical difficulties of life without locomotion came terrible humiliation—the sympathy one might receive today for being handicapped was practically non-existent in the late 1800s.

If movement was not regained quickly after the illness, an inexorable, physical descent would usually follow. When muscles are not being actively enervated by the neurons that control them, they will shrink and waste away. Similarly, the bones these muscles are attached to will suffer. Bones grow as they should when demand is placed upon them from active muscle tension. When muscles develop weakness, the bones will not grow evenly and the sufferer may eventually develop a severely contorted pose we associate with poliomyelitis. The splinting and bracing that was such a popular treatment for decades invariably caused more suffering for those on whom it was practiced. No amount of physical force could prevent the deformities nature would inflict.

Occasionally, paralysis would spread upwards along the spinal cord, and a paralyzed abdomen might result. In the same way, someone's leg might shrivel and grow in an odd direction, paralysis on one side of the lower trunk could—over years of suffering—twist the stoutest human into a knot of flesh and bone. Lesions still further up the column might cause paralysis of one of the arms, even hands. Although these injuries were rare, aggressive splints and braces were applied in hopes the child might maintain some semblance of use with their appendages.

None of these impairments—even if the patients were never to recover from them—were likely to kill. If they were lucky, their legs might be the only limbs affected. If the disease progressed, it would ascend up the spinal cord and affect corresponding muscles. Even with both arms and legs paralyzed, it might still not be enough to end their life directly.

If the damage ascended even higher—thankfully a rare event—it could reach areas that affect breathing. Many who suffered this misfortune could breathe unassisted, but only for a time. The neurons that controlled the diaphragm and intercostal muscles between their ribs would fail to fire. Eventually, expanding their lungs would require more effort than they were capable of, and the air would grow stale as the gas exchange that supplied oxygen ceased. Their mental faculties would remain intact, but respiration would demand complete focus to activate the few muscle fibers that remained under their control. Breathing—an undertaking which just hours earlier had been completely involuntary—would now require an act of God to sustain.

For many of those who struggled to breathe, the Irish physician's 1832 artificial respiration machine would have only prolonged their life. Its hand-operated bellows would have required around-the-clock operation by a team of able-bodied humans, something which most in the 19th century could not afford.

Chapter Nine

Paris Green

THE GYPSY MOTH EGGS HAD HATCHED AT 27 Myrtle Street. They had emerged as caterpillars and were scouring the giant oak trees that surrounded the property for food. While this was happening, another insect invasion was fanning across the country, this time from west to east. The potato beetle, or *Leptinotarsa decemlineata*, is a roundish yellow insect with ten black stripes that run down its back. Its natural habitat had long been the Western United States and Mexico, but in the 1800s as settlers moved across the country, the cultivated potato they brought with them provided a new source of food, and the beetle was able to expand its range eastward.

Its steady march seemed unstoppable and, by 1869, the

voracious insect had reached Ohio. In a desperate attempt to halt its progress, a new pesticide called Paris green was employed. Paris green was an arsenic-based pigment that had been developed in the early 1800s to great acclaim. At that time, there were few options for painters, clothiers, or anyone else who wanted to make something green, so the brilliant emerald hue was tremendously popular and began being used for wallpapers, fabric, toys, and even occasionally, food.

Although it was a favored medicinal ingredient, arsenic had long been known as toxic. Why its use in coloring consumer goods was thought to be safe is unclear, but as a consequence, 19th century literature is replete with stories of death due to poisonings—both accidental and otherwise—from the green color dye and the arsenic it contained. As safer tints arrived on the market, Paris green began to be sold as a powerful pesticide, and its toxicity was thoroughly put to use when the steadfast Potato Beetle began its trek across the country.

Despite the danger of spraying a toxic chemical like arsenic directly onto produce to be consumed by humans, aggressive campaigns to control the potato beetle were undertaken. There was a problem with its application. Paris green, whether dusted onto plants in powder form or sprayed onto them in liquid form, would not adhere to the leaves—the slightest bit of rain or even dew could wash it off. This meant the leaves would only be protected so long as an application stayed dry. And to compound the problem, repeated coatings tended to burn the leaves, ruining the crop they were trying to defend. Striking the right balance between protection from the beetles and destroying the plant—especially when conducted over thousands and thousands of acres—became an impossible task.

By 1874, the potato beetle had reached the Atlantic Coast. Apparently, Paris green had followed with it because a few years later an ominous bit of research was presented at the New York Academy of Medicine by a prominent neurologist, E. C. Seguin. Although the topic had been studied before, he felt compelled to address a growing problem: paralysis following arsenic poisoning. Seguin spent considerable time providing obscure references within the medical literature about the phenomenon, noting a familiar theme:

> *"In lead paralysis the forearms are usually affected (sometimes only one) arsenical paralysis tends to involve all the limbs ; the lower limbs are more affected..."*[10]

Ingested arsenic could occasionally inflame the bowels enough to kill, but it was his recounting of Popov—a Russian scientist who had conducted thorough studies of arsenic poisoning in animals—that should have given anyone listening pause. The results of the post-mortem spinal cord analyses made it clear what was happening:

> *"Arsenic, even in a few hours after its ingestion, may cause distinct lesions of the spinal cord, of the type known as acute central myelitis, or acute poliomyelitis."*[11]

It wasn't just scientists that had noticed. Articles and letters from concerned farmers began to appear in agricultural journals like *Insect Life* and *The Country Gentlemen*.

> *Thanks for Nos. 1 and 2 of "Insect Life." Your publications are*

great public educators and special aids to farmers... A more thorough knowledge of our friends and foes among insects and birds would increase our farm products. We hope you may find out insecticides which are less dangerous to humanity than arsenic. Two cases of serious illness, but not fatal, have occurred in our neighborhood—one from eating strawberries planted alternately with potatoes which had been dusted with Paris green, and the other from eating raspberries adjoining the potato patch, from which the poison had blown. We hope that Congress will make all necessary appropriations for the carrying on of the good work.—[R. Bingham, Camden, N. J., September 22, 1888.

REPLY.— * * *I am glad to get the account of the two cases of poisoning from the treatment of potatoes by Paris green, and agree with you that a less dangerous remedy would be good. With proper care, however, there is very little danger, and in both the instances which you mention the application was evidently very carelessly made.—[September 25, 1888.]*[12]

The arsenic of Paris green may have caused isolated incidents of poisoning—possibly even paralysis—as the potato beetle filed towards the eastern seaboard, but in the confusion of that time, the ability for the ingested poison to paralyze was lost on all but the most astute physicians. The powerful toxicity of the emerald pesticide was considered its strength. Its weaknesses, however, would need to be addressed, and soon—they desperately needed something that would adhere to what it was sprayed on, something that couldn't easily be washed off. The gypsy moths were much hardier than the beetle, and it wasn't the leaves of the potato—resting safely underground—they were after.

Chapter Ten

Boston, 1889

On Sunday, March 11, 1888, unseasonably mild temperatures brought everyone out of their homes in Boston and hinted at the possibility of an early spring. Farmers began to till their fields, and boys and girls enjoyed a pleasant day of running barefoot outside. A light rain began to come down that Sunday night as children returned home. While they fell asleep, an enormous weather system formed off the coast and sent temperatures plummeting. By Monday afternoon rain had turned to snow, and over the next few days, as much as four feet fell in parts of Massachusetts. Everything closed—food was scarce, trains could not run, and life stalled for days as one of the largest blizzards ever recorded in North America pounded

New England.

In Medford, the gypsy moth population that had been steadily growing in the woods behind the houses on Myrtle Street would suffer from the cold. The weather destroyed many of the egg masses stuck to trees and fence posts, so that during the summer their numbers would not be sufficient to sound any alarm. That would change during the next winter of 1888-1889. There would be no great blizzard, and, in fact, there would be very little snow at all. It was an especially mild winter, and although a few determined home owners had been walking their property and removing the brown egg masses for years, it would not be enough. The majority of eggs that had been carefully stashed around Medford would hatch. This time, everyone would notice.

One morning in May of 1889, Medford residents awoke to a nightmare. Brighter-than-usual sun poured in through their bedroom windows, casting them from sleep an hour earlier than was typical. Shielding their eyes from the light, they drew their curtains to reveal a disturbing scene: the leaves were gone on the grand trees outside their homes—completely stripped bare, as if fire had consumed every leaf in sight. The shade the trees had once provided was no more, and now they could clearly see every house on either side of their street.

A block away, a horde of caterpillars were ascending the last remaining oak on their street, searching for food. Within a day, it would be completely destroyed. Homeowners raced down the stairs and into their backyards, confirming their fears—their gardens, their fruit and vegetables, all had been consumed by swarms of the hairy creatures. Once outside, they scraped them with dustpans from the sides of their houses and swept them from their front porches with brooms.

As the sources of food disappeared, millions of hungry caterpillars began crossing Myrtle Street in an attempt to satisfy their voracious appetite. A black, pulsating carpet rippled across the road as passing carriages could do nothing to avoid them. Homeowners tried in vain to destroy them, scraping them into giant barrels of kerosene and burning them by the gallon. It seemed like nothing could stop the onslaught.

Walking down Myrtle Street became impossible, as slipping on the throng of creatures was a constant hazard. The houses themselves were under attack as caterpillars crawled through every gap and crack looking for food. They could be found inside closets and pantries, coat pockets and shoes, under pillows and between the sheets.

It wasn't just Myrtle Street—other pockets of attack emerged across the area. As night fell, the constant sound of a million tiny scissors clipping through the leaves kept anyone from sleeping. The trees would be gone by the morning, and many of the caterpillars would probably be inside the houses before then.

The attack would continue until summer, when the millions of caterpillars would spin their cocoons throughout the town to emerge as moths a week or two later. Although the flying insect's range was limited, they would mate and lay between 500 to 1,000 eggs for each pairing. As authorities toured the destruction on Myrtle Street and the surrounding areas, the devastation was surreal. The thermometer read seventy-five degrees, but the landscape was by all appearances the dead of winter, the carcasses of trees all that remained. Even parts of the houses themselves—steps, porch rails, and siding—had been destroyed as they were cast aside in a frantic search to destroy the insects.

The number of caterpillars which attacked Medford that summer defied belief. As its citizens scoured every square inch of their property, trying to strip the hundreds of spongy brown egg masses coating nearly every vertical surface they could see, they realized their efforts would not be enough. There would not be another Blizzard of 1888 for almost one hundred years, and although the authorities began spraying Paris green aggressively, even that would not be sufficient to stop the gypsy moth's advance.

Chapter Eleven

Boston, 1892

THE GYPSY MOTH CONTINUED ITS MARCH EACH spring, fanning out from Medford and beyond. Trees that were not salvageable were cut down and burned. Other trees were sacrificed in an attempt to remove any temptation for future attack. Home prices in some places plummeted as properties were stripped bare of any and all foliage.

Tireless efforts were undertaken by everyone to slow their progress. Tree trunks were banded with sticky printers ink in hopes of trapping the caterpillars before they reached the leaves above. Gangs of twenty, sometimes thirty, men could be seen spanning the branches of a single tree, meticulously removing any egg masses they could find. At night, fires could be seen from afar as men returned from work and set about destroying what their wives and children had caught during the day.

It was a Sisyphean task even Paris green seemed unable to stop. Arsenic is normally toxic by ingestion. Although contact with skin could poison in some circumstances, its effect as a pesticide worked when the food source of the targeted creature —typically leaves—contained enough of the poison to kill. Whether caterpillars had become immune to its effects, or there were simply too many of them was widely debated. Even after throwing caution to the wind and dousing trees with enough Paris green sure to burn their leaves, the insects carried on, unabated.

By 1892, the moths covered an area over 200 square miles. A "Gypsy Moth Commission" had been formed, and men were hired to work full-time in attempts to control the insect's advance. Police inspected vehicles leaving the area for hitchhiking pests, and the spraying of Paris green increased, despite its apparent futility. A chemist, employed by the commission to develop an insecticide more formidable than Paris green, stumbled onto a new formulation: the arsenic remained, but a new component was added—lead.

The new mixture—dubbed lead arsenate—appeared promising. It was toxic to the caterpillars—that was paramount. Where repeated coatings of Paris green seemed to have little effect on them, lead arsenate killed more readily. It mixed more easily into water and didn't require constant stirring, making its application in the field less troublesome. After it was applied, it left a translucent white coating, allowing operators to determine which areas had already been treated. The foliage to which it was applied seemed to tolerate repeated spraying. A single application of Paris green to fragile foliage might produce "shot holes" in the leaves, but lead arsenate seldom appeared to cause this effect. Somehow, despite the addition of lead, it was gentler to the leaves on which it was sprayed.

The most important trait—besides its increased toxicity—was met with elation by those under attack from the gypsy moth. It was sticky. It clung to that which it was applied and might remain even after a torrential downpour. Lead arsenate had everything one might want in a pesticide. It was a bit more expensive than Paris green, but the ability to use less could make for a better long term investment. Despite its cost, lead arsenate would prove to be a powerful tool in the fight against the gypsy moth. Its negative effects on other living creatures, however—particularly humans—would take decades to register.

Throughout 1892, word spread quickly about the promise of a miraculous new pesticide. Many who'd ignored the earlier warnings of the gypsy moth had already lost everything, but those who lived nearby clearly saw the destruction they could impose. No amount of Paris green or manual disposal appeared to have any effect on the insect's proliferation. The mood was dire, but lead arsenate appeared to offer them a weapon with which they might win.

The ingredients were readily available at any local druggist, and, with the spring of 1893 fast approaching, employees of the commission, farmers, woodsmen, even homeowners, began to fan out from Medford and beyond in a furious attempt to stop the moth's spread. Makeshift sprayers were made by connecting hoses and nozzles to hand-operated water pumps mounted on top of garden barrels. The wheels of carriages were coupled with chains and sprockets to power automatic devices that could propel lead arsenate high into the treetops.

With Medford as its epicenter, a veneer of lead arsenate was dropped onto nearly all living foliage for miles. Carriages rolled down alongside roadways, hoping to form a protective barrier between any insects that happened to escape the perimeter they had established. Homeowners tended their vegetable and fruits, confident the horde would pass them by.

During the summer, the daily vigil for signs of the caterpillar—now clearly recognizable to all—brought mixed signals. The initial reaction was positive. Gone were the massive swarms from Myrtle Street that had carpeted roads and houses, but the insects were still present. Less of them, certainly, but as reports of their whereabouts came filtering back into the Gypsy Moth Commission office, it became obvious the containment zone had been breached.

The lead arsenate was doing its job, but it was evident initial estimates of the moth's advance had been too conservative. The insects had made it far beyond the perimeter, and spraying would need to be increased—if not in volume, then at least in scope.

As winter approached and manual laborers continued scouring tree trunks, fence posts and clapboard siding for gypsy moth eggs, a foreboding article appeared in a November 1893 issue of the widely circulated *Boston Medical and Surgical Journal*. It was called "Is Acute Poliomyelitis Unusually Prevalent This Season?"[13]

Chapter Twelve

Boston, 1893

By this time, poliomyelitis was beginning to appear less often as isolated cases but instead within what they called epidemics. Rather than an infant here or a young boy two towns away, they might discover seven or eight cases of poliomyelitis that either went to the same school or had contacts who did. Although the numbers weren't big enough to qualify as what we might think of as an epidemic, there appeared to be some vector of transmission—invisible to anyone but the most astute observer.

Amidst discussion around the cause of this new disease, its summertime peak was a constant source of speculation. Perhaps it was a meteorological phenomenon, many surmised.

Maybe it was due to flies or mosquitoes that were so prevalent during summer months—perhaps they were carriers of the disease. Whether poliomyelitis involved anything of an infectious nature was unknown, but the way it had begun to surface more frequently amongst small clusters of children convinced many that a bacteria—or possibly a "filterable virus"—was responsible.

In the previous year—1892—the combined hospitals of Boston had seen six cases of poliomyelitis from August to November. The bustling Massachusetts General Hospital saw none. In November 1893, neurologist James Putnam asked in the *Boston Medical and Surgical Journal* if acute poliomyelitis had been unusually prevalent that year. There had been twenty-six cases. Although he seemed relatively non-plussed, it was the largest recorded outbreak of polio in America at the time. In fact, nothing came close to it besides the early reference to the 11 or 12 children suffering from *teething paralysis* in Louisiana in 1841—assumed by modern historians to be polio.

Could the aggressive spraying of lead arsenate have triggered this massive outbreak of "distinct lesions of the spinal cord ... of acute poliomyelitis?"[14] Recall that just a few years earlier, the Russian scientist Popov had poisoned animals with arsenic and documented the hallmark signs of polio in their spinal cords underneath his microscope—sometimes within hours. Later he had been able to conduct an examination on the spinal cord of a man who had died from acute arsenic poisoning, and the results confirmed his animal experiments.

A remarkable coincidence perhaps, but two specific areas were mentioned as contributing several cases of poliomyelitis—the Charlestown and Chelsea districts. Out of all the hundreds of thousands of neighborhoods in the United States, these two were located only a few miles from the epicenter of the frantic spraying in Medford. It's not difficult to imagine these adjacent areas making aggressive attempts to protect their property from the ravages of the gypsy moth that summer.

Another small detail from the article pointed directly towards lead arsenate as the source for at least some of the poliomyelitis:

> *"It is also noteworthy that in some of these epidemics atypical and relatively virulent cases have been unusually common. Again, the occasional occurrence of acute poliomyelitis in conjunction with acute polyneuritis, which is probably always of toxic, and often of infectious origin, bears out this view."*[15]

While poliomyelitis was a relatively new phenomenon for many doctors, *neuritis* was not. Neuritis was a diagnosis assigned to those with pain or sensitivity—sometimes felt as pins, needles, or even numbness because of their nervous system. There were a few things that were known to cause it, but a book on "Peripheral Neuritis," also published in 1893, made clear why acute poliomyelitis and acute polyneuritis were often seen together.

> *(b) Arsenical Paralysis*
>
> *Paralysis is an occasional result of poisoning by arsenic... As a rule the lower extremities are attacked before the upper... Atrophy of the muscles occurs very quickly... Arsenical paralysis is ushered in and accompanied by marked sensory disturbance. The patient complains of severe darting, smarting, burning or rheumatic-like pains in the limbs, and of numbness and tingling in the fingers and*

toes... Quite recently Erlicki and Rybalken examined the nervous system in two cases of arsenical paralysis, and found disease of both the anterior horns and peripheral nerves.[16]

Although modern descriptions of polio don't usually mention skin pain or sensitivity, the best physicians of the day (many of whom were in Boston) would not have thought paralysis and neuritis unusual to see together. Even Putnam himself had authored a paper a few years earlier titled, "On Motor Paralysis and Other Symptoms of Poisoning from Medicinal Doses of Arsenic."[17] At that time, physicians would have been confused by the telltale signs of arsenic poisoning specifically because it was usually caused by their own prescriptions, yet most of those stricken with paralysis and neuritis had taken none. They clearly recognized the danger of their arsenical medicine, but were apparently unaware of the frantic spraying of lead arsenate just outside their office windows.

The reason modern accounts of the polio story have missed this anomaly is not difficult to comprehend. It's a tiny article rarely mentioned amongst other dramatic polio outbreaks. Most descriptions note only the town and number of those stricken: Boston. Twenty-six. A more careful reading of the article suggests it was likely that the poliomyelitis doctors had diagnosed wasn't due to bacteria or viruses, but the newly developed arsenical pesticide sprayed with reckless abandon across the area that spring and summer. The battle to control the moth had claimed its first human victims. Though none had died, the effects of their poliomyelitis might remain for the rest of their lives. The next year would not be so kind.

Chapter Thirteen

Vermont, 1894

It was spring in 1894. Arsenic poisoning was on many people's minds due to an increasing number of deaths from an unlikely source—wallpaper. While those who pointed towards the arsenic often contained within the green dyes of many wall coverings were often ridiculed, other physicians, who had seen the ill effects from living in rooms with this particular kind of wallpaper, began to speak up about its dangers. A chemistry professor from Boston's Harvard University had been measuring urine specimens for signs of arsenic when an especially acute case appeared. This man, who was excreting high amounts of arsenic, did not appear to have any exposure to the usual sources of the metal.

Because he was also excreting significant amounts of copper, the professor suspected Paris green the likely source and said, "We may have, in the free use of Paris green in the field and garden, one explanation of the frequent occurrence of arsenic in the system."[18] While the pesticide had undoubtedly caused health problems in many, it was but a prelude to what would happen later that year to residents of Rutland, Vermont —a small town in the western part of the state. Nestled in a valley between two mountain ranges, Rutland is perforated by a rambling stream of water—Otter Creek—that flows northwards into Lake Champlain.

* * *

The local directory listed Rutland residents only by their address and occupation as telephones would not be common within homes for several years. The back of the directory featured an enticing advertisement from "Story's Kidney and Liver Cure. The remedy of remedies!" Another ad touted "Dark, Clouded, Veined, and Mottled" blue marble, undoubtedly produced by Rutland men employed at quarries throughout the area.

Regardless of the vocation listed by their name within the directory, most Rutland residents spent some of their time growing fruits and vegetables. Steam powered machines were changing the agricultural landscape throughout America, but more affordable gas and diesel powered tractors that would turn small-scale family affairs into enormous commercial operations were yet to come. For now, the men and women that lived along Otter Creek were content tending their smaller farms—rows of blueberries, orchards of apple trees—and selling what they could spare.

While the gypsy moth was making steady gains, it would be a few years before it reached Vermont. Regardless, many in the state were ecstatic about news of a more effective pesticide because they had their own pest to deal with—the codling moth. While not as voracious as their gypsy moth brethren, the codling moth's cuisine was decidedly more personal to many in New England. They didn't prefer leaves as much as they did the fruit itself—particularly pears and apples—a diet which gave the moth its nickname, the "appleworm."

Shortly after winter, local farmers would begin to ready themselves for a long spring of tilling, planting and protecting their crops from the many invaders that could threaten their livelihood. The frequent—and often times unsuccessful—applications of Paris green left much to be desired.

The Rutland druggist may have suggested they purchase materials to make lead arsenate, the miracle pesticide being used to wide acclaim in Massachusetts. Although it had been employed for the past two summers in the areas around Boston, commercial production had not ramped up to fill the demand. Because of this, the correct blend for making the pesticide and its application procedures were still being determined. The amount of water to apply it with—some suggested two pounds of lead arsenate for 50 gallons of water, while others would suggest double, triple, or even quadruple that amount—was another variable that was being established on the fly.

Whatever the recipe called for, its toxicity to humans was not a remote concern. Lead arsenate was remarkably gentle on foliage and could be liberally applied without fear of burning the leaves. Its adhesive property prevented it from easily washing off with rain or dew. These traits had worked to great effect in Boston where the tenacious gypsy moth was destroying every tree in its path.

In Vermont, however, it wasn't trees that needed protection so much as food—fruits and vegetables that were planted in spring and harvested throughout the summer. Lead arsenate appeared to be much more toxic than Paris green and would inevitably be sprayed directly onto produce meant for human consumption. The poliomyelitis that physicians had seen in Boston the previous summer was but a prelude.

Within months, Charles Caverly, a physician and President of the Vermont State Board of Health began hearing accounts from his colleagues of unexplainable "acute nervous disease" in the children of Rutland. More concerning—it was accompanied by paralysis. Throughout the summer and into fall, more reports of illness trickled into his office. By the time he had compiled them all and published his findings in the *Yale Medical Journal*, 123 people would be stricken by this new illness and eighteen of them would die—many of them children.

The outbreak of nervous disease and paralysis in 1894 Rutland, Vermont, is widely considered to be the first epidemic of polio in the United States. A careful examination of the details regarding those who were stricken suggests the answer is more complex.

Chapter Fourteen

Caverly

BY JULY OF 1894, AS THE FIRST produce of the season—boysenberries, potatoes, cherries, and strawberries—began to be harvested, Dr. Charles Caverly began to hear of several children that had been left crippled by a strange disease he was not familiar with. The casualty list would grow throughout the summer and by September 1st, 123 people would be affected—eighteen of them, dead. He was so baffled by the assortment of symptoms and number of victims that he began to collect details in an attempt to deconstruct what might have happened.

Case 4.
Practice of Dr. Fox, Rutland. Boy, 6 years, previous health fair.

> *On two or three occasions had convulsions, presumably due to gastro-intestinal disturbance. Was seized, with convulsions while playing on the street; they continued for nine hours. Moderate fever, rapid pulse, vomiting and rigidity of muscles of the neck and back. No paralysis noted during conscious intervals. Retention of urine during the last three days of illness. Death on the sixth day.*[19]

It is difficult to read the accounts of those who were suffering so horribly that summer of 1894 in Rutland, Vermont. To make matters worse, common medical practices of the day would dictate that strong purgatives be administered with nearly any sickness—usually in the form of mercurial powders. Arsenical tonics such as Fowler's Solution might also be employed. Because of this, when someone of that time period presented with an illness, and a few days later showed signs of paralysis, one must consider that the medical treatments they likely received might have been a part of the problem. Regardless, a careful examination of the cases presented by Dr. Caverly's thorough documentation of the epidemic does not align with a modern definition of polio.

Regarding the six-year-old boy, a rapid pulse, fever, and vomiting might be consistent with the initial infection of the poliovirus. Convulsions, however, are not. At its worst, polio might present as muscle weakness—if not outright paralysis. The sudden, violent contraction of muscles exhibited by convulsions are not considered indicative of polio, but instead acute lead or arsenic poisoning.

The rigid neck and back the boy experienced might point to polio *or* poisoning. Either way, the fact he died without showing any signs of paralysis whatsoever would make for an odd polio diagnosis nowadays. Death from polio typically occurs as the mechanisms that support respiration fail. This is not a sudden, catastrophic event, but a gradual process with ancillary effects that would have clearly pointed to asphyxiation as the cause.

The gastro-intestinal disturbances that appeared to trigger the onset of the boy's convulsions are typical of metal poisoning, and one can only hope these ailments didn't provoke the administration of metallic medicines.

> *Case 32.*
>
> *Practice of Dr. Marshall, Wallingford. Woman 21 years. Married and one child of 16 months. Apparent cause fatigue from nursing sick child. First had head- and backache. Pulse 80, temperature 98.6°. On third day pulse 100, temperature 103.5°. Some opisthotonos; bowels regular; urine, 2 pints in twenty-four hours. No albumin, no sugar. Urticarial blotches on the body. During the next three or four days temperature ranged from 100.5° to 102°, pulse about 100. Was unable to speak or swallow. Answered questions by moving the head; in no pain. Sixth day temperature 98.6°; pulse 60. Remained in this condition five days. On the eleventh day complained of severe pain in the stomach, and neck became rigid; pulse 100, temperature 98.6°. During the next two days pulse became very irregular. Complained of severe pain in the right side of the head and right eye. Died at the end of the second week.*[20]

The twenty-one-year-old woman's symptoms are remarkably unlike a modern interpretation of paralytic polio. Being unable to speak or swallow is indicative of acute cranial nerve palsies—a possible, but uncommon, complication of what is called *bulbar polio*. The urticarial blotches on the body —red hives that break out on the skin—are not so ambiguous—they have no association with a poliovirus infection but are strongly associated with arsenic poisoning.[21]

Like the boy mentioned in "Case 4," this woman's initial illness was possibly treated with mercuric or arsenical medicine. Whatever caused her initial suffering was likely lost amongst the growing constellation of misery. Her complaints of severe pain in the right side of her head and behind her right eye are consistent with the pathology seen in autopsies of those who died from acute mercury poisoning.

Her death came after nearly two weeks of increased suffering—again without any sign of paralysis or breathing difficulties. Whether a true poliovirus infection would have caused her particular symptoms is unlikely. The fact she was experiencing hives on her skin clearly points towards the likelihood of acute poisoning by either arsenic or lead, possibly both.

> *Case 116.*
>
> *Practice of Dr. Swift, Pittsford. Boy, 4 years, Italian. Taken with headache, drowsiness and slow hobbling pulse. Little fever. After four days developed strabismus. Improved speedily and at the end of four days was apparently well. Three days later, after playing too hard, had a return of the original symptoms. Headache, drowsiness, no fever, pulse 45. In two days from this time had a convulsion and speedily died.*[22]

The four-year-old boy mentioned in case 116 is similar to many others that died that summer. The prototypical stages of poliovirus infection would later be recognized as initially a trivial illness—fever, headache, and possibly a stomach ache—followed several days later by paralysis, typically starting in the legs. While the boy recovered from his initial symptoms, rather than developing paralysis, he began having convulsions and quickly died. Neither convulsions or a sudden death with no sign of paralysis would suggest polio.

Amongst the eighteen whose lives were claimed, seven of them showed no paralysis at all. Other symptoms, for sure, but a very odd phenomenon if the 1894 outbreak is to be considered a polio epidemic. A look through the other cases that Caverly mentions reveals similar incongruities. Many exhibited affections of the skin or extreme sensitivity—the same polyneuritis that accompanied the previous summer's outbreak in Boston—symptoms which point directly towards arsenic poisoning rather than the poliovirus.

One of the Rutland physicians who treated nineteen of those who were sickened gave additional testimony that called into question what role medicine itself may have had in their suffering. Dr. H. L. Newell recounted one of the two fatal cases that he had attended:

> *In this case I saw the child on Sunday and it had an attack of indigestion to all appearances, slight fever, committing and diarrhea. I prescribed for the child and the next day I was sent word that the child was better and I would not have to see it. The next day, Tuesday, being at the next neighbors, the mother called me in. The child had some fever and little diarrhea. I left some medicine with directions that if the child did not gain to let me know. I heard nothing more about the case until a week after that,*

but the next Tuesday I was called in haste and found the child in a collapse and apparently dying. I put it in a hot bath and the child revived a little but had convulsions and lived but twenty-four hours.[23]

The medicine Dr. Newell left with the child's mother was most likely mercuric in nature. Mercury was known to be toxic but, regardless, the dosage was often increased if the patient's health did not improve. Oliver Wendell Holmes, who penned the lyrics to the 1869 *Hymn of Peace*, detested many of these medicines so much he was quoted as saying if a ship-load of them "could be sunk to the bottom of the sea, it would be all the better for mankind and all the worse for the fishes."[24]

Many of the children in Vermont developed vomiting, a fever or diarrhea before their paralysis, and we can be sure that —like the boy who Dr. H. L. Newell described—they were administered mercury- or arsenic-containing medicine. A broader statement Caverly made regarding many of the children who had suffered from the illness should give anyone additional skepticism as to the role of poliovirus in Rutland that summer:

It was not infrequently remarked by physicians practicing in this valley at the time of this epidemic, that the usual diseases of children were accompanied with exaggerated nervous symptoms. Headache, convulsions and delirium were common.[25]

Beside convulsions, delirium is not something mentioned alongside polio infections. Delusions and incoherence of speech do frequently accompany metal poisoning—as evidenced by the fevered construction of asylums and fainting rooms during the 1800s. Perhaps it was an especially hot July and August, and the sick children acutely felt the effects of overheating. A more plausible explanation—it was an especially hot season, and the sick children had been enjoying their fill of fresh apples or strawberries.

Caverly himself admitted confusion as to whether the outbreak was indeed polio, as he realized "some of the commonest symptoms seen in our epidemic were entirely foreign to this disease as long described."[26] While the convulsions, skin conditions, and polyneuritis so prevalent that summer may not have been enough to convince physicians that the recent introduction of lead arsenate was a plausible culprit, its possible role should be obvious to any modern reader.

But another part of the story—a small piece, often neglected—leaves no doubt as to whether pesticides were playing a role in the "acute nervous disease" that had struck down residents of Vermont that summer. It wasn't just people that had been afflicted with nervous disorders—it was also animals.

Chapter Fifteen

Animals

DR. CHARLES L. DANA, A PHYSICIAN WHO was directly involved with the 1894 Vermont epidemic, forwarded portions of brain and spinal cord from one of the victims to the Carnegie Laboratory for examination. The results were unmistakable to a scientist who analyzed the tissue:

> *Microscopic examination shows an acute poliomyelitis of the lumbar part of the cord... I feel the greatest possible confidence that the disease is in most cases a true anterior poliomyelitis.*[27]

The victim in this case was not a human, but a chicken. The spinal cord of at least one of twelve horses who had succumbed to paralysis of the lower limbs was also examined and pronounced to resemble poliomyelitis. Countless dogs suffered a similar fate. All over the valley around Rutland, animals—like their human counterparts—had suffered from paralysis in their hind legs, sometimes death.

Physicians didn't know it at the time, but the poliovirus is incapable of paralyzing nearly any animal on the planet. Rabbits, guinea pigs, mice, and other animals were purposefully injected with what was assumed to contain the microbe responsible for paralysis, but none of them seemed to be affected by it. By chance, the procedure was tried successfully on two Old World monkeys—a fortuitous stroke of luck in the study of the poliovirus, because even New World monkeys are apparently immune to its neurotropic effects. One of the monkeys developed paralysis resembling the effects of poliomyelitis and later died. The other showed no paralysis, but also died. Upon examination, both of their spinal cords appeared to demonstrate the lesions characteristic of the disease.

In 1908,[28] the results of this experiment were presented to a rapt group of scientists and physicians in Vienna, Austria, who had assumed the cause of poliomyelitis would be discovered to be a single pathogen. While the mode of transmission and the route of infection were still unknown, those in attendance were no doubt thrilled when the photographs of spinal cord lesions from the two monkeys were displayed. At long last, they had their suspect for what was causing recent epidemics of infantile paralysis.

With this information in mind, it might appear that the scientists who analyzed the dead chicken and horse from

Vermont were mistaken. But as they peered through their microscopes, they simply reported what they had seen: lesions in the grey matter of the spinal cord of the animals—what was officially called poliomyelitis.

This wasn't the first time animals had died from poliomyelitis. Just two years earlier in 1892, M. Roger published a paper in the Pasteur Institute journal describing how he had injected rabbits with modified *streptococcus* bacteria and they developed paralysis in their posterior extremities. They died within a few days and upon examination

> *...showed a muscular atrophy at the site for degeneration, with formation of vacuoles in the ganglion cells of the anterior horns of the cord, an anterior poliomyelitis simulating the pathologic alterations of infantile paralysis.*[29]

It wasn't just streptococcus. Others were able to create poliomyelitis in rabbits using *E. coli* and *Staphylococcus aureus* bacteria.

When a modern reader hears the term *polio*, they inevitably envision paralysis caused by a specific thing—the poliovirus. When it was first discovered, this virus was thought to be the sole microbe responsible for poliomyelitis and was consequently named *poliovirus*. Although direct experimentation was not typically conducted on humans, it was eventually discovered that the poliovirus could indeed paralyze. It has an affinity for replicating in nervous tissue, and the resulting inflammation can apparently cause the lesions of poliomyelitis.

But humans can also be paralyzed by other viruses—not

just the poliovirus. It was later discovered that *coxsackievirus*, *echovirus* and other enteroviruses such as *D68* could also cause poliomyelitis and its ensuing paralysis. The symptoms may appear identical to that of the poliovirus, and even a post-mortem examination of the victim's spinal cord might be unable to distinguish a difference.

These facts suggest a reality that will no doubt confuse the modern reader: Poliomyelitis can be caused by many different things. In humans, there are at least several viruses which can replicate in neural tissue and cause poliomyelitis. Numerous bacteria in animals can trigger the same results. And to complicate matters, recall Popov's experiments which created the hallmark signs of poliomyelitis in creatures he had poisoned with arsenic. All of them—under the right conditions—could cause examples of poliomyelitis that were indistinguishable from one another, even under a microscope.

Unfortunately, after the 1909 presentation in Vienna, the die was cast. Amongst the group of highly esteemed scientists, their quest to locate a single cause was judged to have been a success. Poliomyelitis, it would appear, was caused by a virus—a pathogen so small it couldn't be seen by their most powerful microscopes and could easily pass through their most delicate filters.

After that year, poliomyelitis research becomes more difficult for the modern historian. Before then, Vermont's Dr. Caverly and many others dutifully cataloged the minutiae of each outbreak of poliomyelitis with a blind eye as to its cause and effect, with little to no prejudice. After 1909, case descriptions would become narrower and symptoms that were not in keeping with a viral infection were left out. Animals that had become paralyzed or died within the epidemics would eventually no longer be mentioned. These phenomena did not go away, but were simply overlooked in a tragically human attempt to make sense of a horrible situation. Their eagerness to understand the nature of poliomyelitis would inadvertently narrow their focus at a time when it should have been expanded.

* * *

In 1895, just months after Caverly had reported on the epidemic of poliomyelitis in Rutland, Vermont, a physician in Boston offered his thoughts on the confusing source of the disease. Neurologist James Putnam, who had authored the 1893 article, "Is Acute Poliomyelitis Unusually Prevalent This Season?" would pose a question that would be even more poignant if asked today, almost 125 years later.

> *It is not impossible that we group, clinically, under the name of poliomyelitis, several affections which might in strictness be separated; or, in other words, that several different poisons are liable to affect the anterior horns of the spinal cord, exciting results which, though in the main alike, may differ in detail.*[30]

Poliomyelitis did, in fact, consist of "several affections" rather than the lone virus a vaccine began to be developed for. It was not just the poliovirus, but many other sources—a growing number of sources, actually. This seemingly benign oversight would cause not only confusion for millions, but the suffering and death of many others who later assumed they were safeguarded from the single causative agent of poliomyelitis when, in fact, they may have been protected from only one of its many causes.

As the crisp autumn mornings of Vermont faded away and winter approached, the mysterious paralysis and other nervous ailments of Rutland's children disappeared. Other illnesses of childhood—typhoid, cholera, and summer diarrhea—were still a bigger concern for parents, but the menace of a new disease which had no explanation or cure began to loom large in the minds of the physicians and scientists who tried to untangle it.

Chapter Sixteen

Browntail

In retrospect, it would be easy to place the origin of the 1894 Vermont outbreak squarely upon the toxic effects of lead arsenate, introduced just a year or so earlier: the sickened animals—incapable of developing polio infections—who probably ate freely from the sprayed fruit as it dropped onto the ground amongst the orchards they inhabited; the children, particularly vulnerable, who began to consume produce as it was harvested beginning in early summer. Many symptoms listed by Caverly—polyneuritis, urticarial blotches, death with no paralysis—appear to be unrelated to polio but instead point towards arsenic or lead poisoning.

These same patterns would be repeated over the next few

years in smaller epidemics: summer, children, often boys, animals—symptoms that are not in keeping with a modern definition of polio. Even the rural landscape of Vermont would serve as a template for future poliomyelitis outbreaks. For the time being, cities appeared remarkably immune to large epidemics.

* * *

In 1897, Massachusetts began to suffer the effects of yet another invasive insect—the browntail moth. The gypsy moth was slowly migrating farther away from its humble beginnings on Myrtle Street in Medford and a new predator had rushed in behind it. Despite their best efforts to contain the gypsy moth, the insect had continued to spread and was beginning to show incredible resilience to the effects of arsenic poisoning. Tests were conducted, and many of the caterpillars could survive ingesting amounts of arsenic ten to fifteen times higher than what was thought to be lethal. The limitations of laboratory study were becoming obvious and so concentrations of the pesticide were ramped up in a frantic attempt to stop the creature.

With the addition of the browntail moth, the codling and gypsy moths presented a threat so ominous many threw caution to the wind and began to spray with an intensity guaranteed to cause problems. Crews slashed and burned trees and brush in an attempt to create a fire-break the insects could not cross. If landowners did not consent to the destruction of their property in this way, giant wagons would swoop in and cover the foliage in the sticky film of lead arsenate.

Mechanized labor allowed unheard-of efficiency as farms began to specialize in fewer crops and larger tracts of land. An industry was born to serve commercial farming, and companies began to aggressively advertise the potential of their lead arsenate. Within years, the pesticide gained widespread adoption by growers across the country, eager to maximize the yields of their crop and blinded to the potential dangers of produce coated in a mixture of lead and arsenic that—by design —would not easily wash off.

Other invasive species became targets, such as the recently imported cattle tick, which was the cause of much death and destruction to livestock across the South. To combat the devastation, animals were marched through long ditches filled with water and arsenic—known as cattle dips—their heads forced underwater to immerse them completely in the pesticides. Unfortunate farmhands were sometimes stationed directly in the dip, standing all day in the arsenic-infested water to aid in herding the reluctant cattle onward.

Investigators soon discovered that arsenic residues could be found on "peas, carrots, apples, mushrooms, pears, rice, beef, veal, mackerel, eggs, potatoes, spinach, white beans, cabbage, lettuce, dried peas, dried fruits."[31] The industry manufacturing lead arsenate began to hire scientists to conduct studies to determine the safety of their products. Unsurprisingly, their reports minimized the dangers of exposure to the pesticide and even belittled the public's growing concern about the presence of the metal in their lives.

A tongue-in-cheek editorial written by the editors of the *Medical Record* mocked those concerned by the potential toxicity of arsenic, stating

> *the condition of our esteemed and interesting colleagues of Massachusetts... having passed safely through disquieting exacerbations of homeopathy, mind-cure, Ibsenism,*[i] *and physical research, the profession has been brought up sharply with an attack of arseniophobia... the evidence seems to accumulate in favor of the view that in Boston rural arsenic poisoning is an infectious disease... In fact there seems to be an appalling possibility that Massachusetts is being systematically poisoned by an inoculable, malignantly infective, and extremely prevalent form of arsenical poisoning. We rejoice to learn that the Legislature and State Board of Health are at work upon the matter.*

Despite the public's increasing worry about the possible effects of lead arsenate—and efforts within the government to create meaningful regulation around its use—the pesticide would quickly become the most popular defense against insects within years.

Perhaps not coincidentally, it became clear that outbreaks of poliomyelitis were on the rise. Within the entire United States, the period of 1885-1889 produced only 23 cases of suspected poliomyelitis. The Rutland, Vermont outbreak pushed the 1890-1894 period to 151 cases amongst what are described as four separate epidemics. The 1895-1899 period contained 23 epidemics and would soon explode to 25 between 1905-1909 with over eight-thousand people suffering the effects of poliomyelitis.[32]

In 1907, New York City suffered its first epidemic—unusual at the time for an urban area. Massachusetts, Minnesota,

---

i. *A philosophical exploration, of sorts.*

Wisconsin, and Iowa saw outbreaks in 1908, and the next year would add Pennsylvania, the District of Columbia, Virginia, and Connecticut to the list.[33] It was clear this once unknown malady was becoming a major problem.

With increasing amounts of arsenic and lead—not to mention aluminum and mercury—foisted upon the public at this time, it would be easy to place the blame of poliomyelitis entirely upon these toxic metals. But despite the infected animals and decidedly un-polio-like symptoms, there appeared to be something else going on—something infectious about the way the disease was spreading.

Chapter Seventeen

Epidemic

AS EPIDEMIOLOGISTS ATTEMPTED TO MAP THE ADVANCE of poliomyelitis, confusion reigned supreme. For years, the nature of the disease had eluded them—was it due to an infectious agent? Was it contagious? How did it spread? Was it transmissible by an insect such as a mosquito or the house fly? Why were children targeted so often? Why the summer and not the spring or fall?

After the 1909 Vienna presentation demonstrated how a virus could be successfully passed from the spinal cord of someone who had died with poliomyelitis into monkeys, the answers to these questions would become even more difficult to ascertain. If poliomyelitis was due to an infectious agent, why was its spread so unsystematic? As a 1910 public health report stated, "If the disease has been disseminated from New York along routes of travel, it is hard to understand why it has progressed so irregularly, skipping wide areas of thickly settled country, and why it has spread so slowly, becoming epidemic in the District of Columbia, for example, three years subsequent to the epidemic in New York."[34]

Knowing that many cases of poliomyelitis appear to be arsenic and/or lead poisoning should have provided a bit of consolation for the scattershot nature of its spread. But a look at the cases of poliomyelitis epidemics suggests there *was* in fact some kind of infectious vector to its spread—something more than simply a random chance poisoning from pesticides.

In Rutland, Vermont, the dead animals and neuritis provide little doubt their suffering had much to do with lead arsenate, yet there were others who did not suffer like this—their symptoms were more in keeping with a modern description of polio. And although a local druggist may have provided inappropriate instructions for the formulation of lead arsenate that summer, it seems highly unlikely that no one else throughout the state of Vermont made the same mistake—the epidemic was limited to a group of people located up and down Otter Creek, all within 15 miles of each other.

If it had been a city like Boston or New York, one might suppose a single vendor had sold all of the victims food or milk contaminated with toxic amounts of arsenic. People were beginning to suspect these things as possible sources of the disease precisely because a few epidemics—not all of them—shared a common produce or milk supplier, both of which were known to occasionally contain dangerous amounts of arsenic.

But the epidemics were happening mainly in the rural countryside, where pesticides were aggressively sprayed, and fruits, vegetables, and milk were more likely home-grown.

Caverly noted that very few families within the 1894 outbreak had more than one victim—a strange phenomenon for an infectious disease *or* pesticide poisoning amongst a group of people who most likely ate and drank from the same sources. He also highlighted the fact that although many cases occurred along Otter Creek, the residents of houses that were closest to the water appeared to have been spared any suffering. As he plotted the location of the victims and their day to day interactions, a few connecting threads would materialize only to disappear upon further inspection. Other epidemics would present similarly frustrating gaps in understanding the transmission of a potential virus.

Eventually, physicians began to believe that for every person who developed poliomyelitis, many others had developed the viral infection responsible for it—without showing any paralysis, possibly without presenting any symptoms of sickness at all. These *asymptomatic carriers* were thought to be the missing link in the fractured outbreak maps and the method by which the virus was traveling. Although scientists were beginning to believe that all of poliomyelitis was caused by a single pathogen, why some developed an infection with no apparent side effects—while others might perish from it—would continue to torment physicians for years.

* * *

In 1910, sixteen years after the original outbreak, Vermont suffered another epidemic of poliomyelitis, and Dr. Caverly was ready to document as much as he could. Again, the preponderance of cases involved boys under five, and amongst the 52 cases of paralysis, only five of them didn't involve their legs in some way.

There was a new demographic this time, however. While the 1894 epidemic had also affected horses, chickens, and dogs, the 1910 episode involved a new paralytic disease in calves and pigs. Caverly may have been unaware of the 1909 report documenting how Old World monkeys appeared to be the only animals capable of being infected with the poliovirus, but regardless, he could not deny what he saw and documented it clearly:

> *It is of course regrettable that neither of these instances of disease in the lower animals was discovered in time to have adequate pathological or bacteriological examinations made. They emphasize, however, the facts: that the disease affects lower animals, that it occurs in connection with the disease in the human family, and that there are good prima facie reasons for thinking there may be a common cause for cases in man and the lower animals, and that it maybe communicated from animals to man and vice versa.*[35]

Caverly wasn't the only one confused by the continuance of animal paralysis and death associated with poliomyelitis outbreaks. Others would note this dilemma and struggle to square a single causative agent against the assortment of sufferers—and symptoms. Perhaps physicians—eager to point the blame away from anything resembling their own medicines—were too quick to embrace the poliovirus as the lone cause of poliomyelitis. Either way, while scientists of the time felt they were zeroing in on the mystery behind infantile paralysis, a modern reading—taken from a 50,000 foot view—reveals they were getting further away.

Chapter Eighteen

Anatomy

THE POLIOVIRUS, LIKE MANY OTHER ENTEROVIRUSES, THRIVES within the intestines. Although it might be found nearly anywhere on the skin or mucosal tissue—such as the lining of the nose or tonsils—replication within the gut is where it can grow into the millions. Because enteroviruses proliferate within the intestines, their transmission from human to human appears to happen mainly via what is pleasantly described as the *fecal-oral route*. This means that most people do not become infected through person-to-person contact, sneezing, or other airborne transmission methods but rather through ingesting water, food, or anything else which might carry traces of fecal matter contaminated with a virus.

This may not sound like a common occurrence. In First World countries, with modern sanitation and hygiene practices in place, it is thankfully rare. In less civilized areas of the world, it can be an every day occurrence. Even in countries where open, public defecation is stigmatized, the practice of creating separation between pit latrines and drinking water sources are often ignored.

Because of this, water supplies inevitably may become contaminated with fecal material—either through underground aquifers that unknowingly connect wells with latrines, or simply through runoff from old latrines that were not emptied or covered correctly. Pit latrines will only work for smaller population densities—eventually a more advanced system of pipes, pumps, and sewage treatment plants are necessary. In a sparsely populated area, the likelihood of ingesting an enterovirus is low, but in more crowded conditions, the ability for humans to successfully maintain separation between water and sewage becomes much more challenging.

The fear of illness from contaminated water supplies is nearly foreign to many, but there are millions of parents and their children who face the threat of an enterovirus every time they take a sip of water. If an infection takes hold, the victim might experience something as simple as a cold or diarrhea to life-threatening illnesses such as aseptic meningitis or sepsis. While man has known about the need for clean drinking water, this battle of gut versus germ has been fought for time eternal. For thousands of years, enteroviruses seemed incapable of causing problems in the central nervous system, but in the late 1800s, enterovirus infections began to be associated with paralysis.

* * *

It has been said that seventy-percent of the immune system resides in the gut. While the blood and brain both have their own brand of pathogen-fighting white blood cells, the intestine reigns supreme in its remarkable ability to protect the body from the many foreign invaders that inevitably hitch a ride along the food and drink ingested each day. This protection is important because many of the enteroviruses, such as the coxsackievirus or D68, can also proliferate amongst the neuronal cells of the central nervous system.

Many viruses and bacteria are relatively innocuous outside nervous tissue. It is only once they pierce the skin they become dangerous. *Clostridium tetani*, the bacteria responsible for tetanus, is so common that it is not even tested for—it is often assumed that someone exhibiting the symptoms of a possible tetanus infection is likely to have the bacteria whether their nervous system has been infected with it or not. On the skin, the bacteria is harmless. If it gets into the nervous system, it can replicate along the neuronal cell pathways and cause muscle spasms severe enough to break bones. Similarly, the rabies virus is a deadly threat if the skin is punctured and it's able to gain entry into the nervous system. Nearly anywhere else, the virus is benign.

How and why enteroviruses get past the herculean efforts of the intestinal immune system and into the central nervous system is possibly the biggest mystery of all things polio-related. With tetanus and rabies, there is a traumatic puncture wound that can introduce the bacteria or virus directly into the nervous system at the site of the injury. With an enterovirus infection like the poliovirus, there is no such mechanism—yet the pathogen is apparently able to gain entry directly into the spinal cord.

After years of false starts in researching the nature of a poliovirus infection, it was eventually discovered that the pathogen is occasionally able to breach the intestines and gain entry into the blood stream where the body's white blood cells mount an attack and generate enough antibodies that the poliovirus infection will eventually clear.

But even that is not enough to cause paralysis—the virus still needs to gain entry into the spinal cord itself. This may seem like a trivial effort once the virus has breeched the blood supply, but the nature of most poliomyelitis cases presents a thorny problem: Why are the lesions so frequently located at the bottom of the spinal cord, where the legs are affected?

Michael Underwood's "Debility of the Lower Extremities" had first described the phenomenon in 1796, and its predilection for paralysis of the legs has continued to this day. Why would this be? The spinal cord is supplied with blood from three arteries that run from the brain down towards the bottom, plus a set of arteries for each vertebrae that branch off the enormous thoracic aorta that curves downwards from the heart towards the pelvis. In short, the spinal cord is well served by redundant blood supplies—from the top down and from multiple branches all the way down—arteries that have no prejudice or ability to filter certain bacteria or viruses.

Because of this elaborate blood supply, the lesions of poliomyelitis would seem to have an equal chance of developing anywhere along the spinal cord, yet they rarely develop anywhere except the specific area that controls the legs — at the very bottom. Even in cases of animal poliomyelitis that were created with purposeful arsenic poisoning within a laboratory setting, it was the hind legs of the creatures that often suffered the most dramatic paralysis.

Initially, researchers were perplexed and thought that coagulation of blood in specific locations might be preventing the injurious agent—whatever it was—from reaching other areas of the cord. This line of research was quickly abandoned and there were few alternate explorations. While this anatomical mystery should have created a determined search for its cause, it still persists and appears to be accepted as something science will never understand.

An additional quirk of poliomyelitis—the tendency for *anterior,* or front side, lesions of the spinal cord—may provide a clue for what is happening. Occasionally, lesions will appear on the back half of the cord, causing extreme sensitivity but, more often than not, it is the front side of the cord, a phenomenon which can cause motor nerve disruption and paralysis. The rear side of the spinal cord is served by two *posterior spinal arteries* while the front has only one *anterior spinal artery.* If blood flow had much to do with the introduction of paralyzing pathogens into the central nervous system, one might be inclined to believe the posterior spinal cord would receive the brunt of damage.

A quick look at an anatomical model of the human body presents an intriguing hypothesis. In an infant, the spinal cord is nearly the same length as the spine. As the baby develops, the spine and its vertebrae grow much more than the cord itself. Once adulthood is reached, the spine and its vertebrae are fully grown and the spinal cord ends much higher than infants—somewhere around the 2nd lumbar vertebra.

The result of this phenomenon is that for infants, a significant section of their spinal cord sits directly behind their intestines, where the assault from both enteroviruses and ingested metals or pesticides often occurs. As the body grows into adulthood, the location of the intestines moves farther down and away from the end of the spinal cord.

To accept that an ingested toxin such as arsenic—which is known to cause poliomyelitis—could enter the blood stream and circulate throughout the body and somehow traverse the entire spinal cord without causing any damage except for the very bottom section—is a difficult ask. The same could be said for any of the enteroviruses capable of causing paralysis. Knowing that ingested metals, pesticides, or enterovirus likely started their journey a few centimeters away in the intestine makes it more difficult to believe this circuitous, fortuitous route could happen over and over throughout the late 1800s and early 1900s.

Certain pesticides and metals are known to negatively affect the cell membrane function of organs in which they lodge.[36] Perhaps the ingested lead arsenate in 1894, Vermont, was so toxic it was able to wreck the intestinal linings of its victims and migrate into the nerves or blood supply situated directly behind. While this may seem like a fanciful hypothesis, the prevailing notion that infection happens through the blood poses many more problems given the extremely selective location so often damaged.

Additional details regarding poliomyelitis infection may support this hypothesis. The way in which adult spinal cords are located further away from their intestines than children might explain why adults are often spared—and why babies appear so uniquely vulnerable to the effects of *infantile* or *teething paralysis*. If poliomyelitis was universally the result of a viral or bacterial infection, one could argue that adults had successfully developed immunity to these pathogens whereas infants had not—a view which begs an obvious question—why were adults able to develop immunity without harm in the first place? But poliomyelitis could be triggered by many things besides pathogens and, no matter the source—microbes, metals, or pesticides—children appeared much more susceptible than adults.

Another frequent event associated with the onset of poliomyelitis was over-exertion, playing too hard or "overheating." Caverly noted in 1894 that of the 37 cases where an apparent cause was stated, "overheating" was mentioned 24 times.[37] This association would continue well into the 1950s, visible on "Polio Precaution" posters that were placed in nearly every school and doctor's office: Don't mix with new groups. Don't get overtired. Don't get chilled. But do keep clean.

If ingested metals or pesticides are capable of creating cell membrane dysfunction, perhaps the agitation of extreme physical activity maximized the chance for toxins to work their way out of the intestines and into adjacent spinal cord tissue. That the lesions of poliomyelitis are so often on the front side of the spinal cord—even though blood flows freely to all areas—may convince some their anatomical proximity to the intestine is no coincidence.

It is possible that an interaction between ingested metals *and* an enterovirus infection offers a mechanism by which many formerly trivial viruses were able to reach the central nervous system. In the intestine of someone with few pesticides or metals, an enterovirus infection might appear as a common cold—an insignificant sickness that would come and go in a day or two. Even if an adult's gut was wrecked from medicinal mercury or from consuming fruit coated in lead arsenate, an enterovirus infection might escape the confines of the intestines but never make it all the way into their spinal cord a few inches away.

But in a child whose spinal cord was nestled directly against their intestines, mercuric teething powders or lead arsenate might combine with a simultaneous enterovirus infection to create the perfect opportunity for an otherwise innocuous virus to do serious damage. In a gut compromised from chronic metal or pesticide toxicity, many of the enteroviruses that infect millions of people each day may gain the ability to cross over into the nervous system and create the lesions of poliomyelitis.

It turns out the poliovirus may have been responsible for some of the paralysis in Rutland, Vermont, after all. But it did not act alone—it needed help from something capable of disrupting the normal protective function of the intestinal immune system. With the introduction of lead arsenate just two years earlier and 150 miles away, it seems likely the quest of the Vermont farmer to protect their produce from the codling moth—and perhaps even the growing threat of the gypsy moth—may have come at the worst possible time.

Chapter Nineteen

Spray, O Spray

It was 1914 and the wonders of lead arsenate mesmerized those who grew food for a living. Everyone was encouraged to coat their fruits and vegetables with the wonder pesticide. Farmers who didn't were frowned upon by their neighbors—perhaps an early harbinger of the epidemiologist's favorite construct, herd immunity. By the end of the 19th century, many states had passed laws that required farmers to spray their cops with pesticides. If for some reason they were unable to, they would need to pay to have it done. Additional penalties were employed for farmers caught transporting invasive species within the food they sold.

Entomologists of the day—formerly thought of as grown

men running through fields with butterfly nets—were no doubt thrilled with their recently discovered power and authority. Lead arsenate was now a mandatory application, and the economic costs of runaway invasive species such as the gypsy or codling moths were beginning to be understood.

A hymn to the newfound riches to be had with the new pesticide may have not been necessary, but nevertheless, this paean likely provided confidence to any farmer that may have doubted the safety of his chemical applications:

Spray, farmers, spray with care,
Spray the apple, peach and pear;
Spray for scar, and spray for blight,
Spray, O spray, and do it right.

Spray the scale that's hiding there,
Give the insect all a share;
Let your fruit be smooth and bright,
Spray, O spray, and do it right.

Spray your grapes, spray them well,
Make first class what you've to sell,
The very best is none too good,
You can have it, if you would.

Spray your roses, for the slug,
Spray the fat potato bug;
Spray your cantaloupes, spray them thin,
You must fight if you would win.

Spray for blight, and spray for rot,
Take good care of what you've got;

Spray, farmers, spray with care,
Spray, O spray the buglets there.[38]

And so spray they did. No pest—invasive or not—was safe. Everything was treated with liberal amounts of lead arsenate. Many farmers still turning rows with plow and mule spent their hard earned money not on a mechanical tractor but instead, a mechanical sprayer from which they could drench their produce. As this new pesticide became the go-to method of insect control, Paris green would begin to be marketed as rat poison—an interesting application considering it had been dusted liberally on fruits and vegetables for years.

Although the sticky quality of lead arsenate worked as advertised, overzealous farmers would augment its adhesive nature by adding casein or oil, turning it into a gummy substance that was unlikely to be removed by anything—rain or man. Studies would later confirm this as comparisons between apples that had been sprayed two days previous and two *months* previous showed little appreciable difference in the amount of arsenic they contained.

At the same time, spraying technology improved, and the cost of lead arsenate began to go down. Farmers rejoiced at their increased productivity, and customers were no doubt elated at the beautiful "fruit, smooth and bright." With the admonition to "Spray, O Spray" coming at them from every angle, it's little wonder that much of the nation's food supply became contaminated with potentially harmful amounts of arsenic and lead.

Reports of children killed by arsenic poisoning began to surface, and authorities—who had worked tirelessly to enforce the mandatory application of pesticides—blamed the deaths on improper spraying techniques by reckless farmers. Scientists financed through agricultural funding wrote thinly-veiled puff pieces for the wonders of lead arsenate. Others made bold claims about the hundreds of apples one would have to eat in order to become poisoned. J.W. Summers, a congressman and physician—from the apple-friendly state of Washington—boasted that no one could produce an "acute or chronic case of arsenic poisoning resulting from the use of apples or pears."

The battle for public opinion over the safety of lead arsenate began to play out in newspapers and magazine articles throughout the country. Because arsenic was still being used as a popular medicinal treatment, it was difficult for whistleblowers to argue that consuming even lesser amounts on food was more dangerous. A little known study was published around that time that might've changed people's minds.

* * *

Much of the early testing of lead arsenate toxicity was conducted on apples—the most popular fruit at the time. Apples had a smooth skin that allowed lead arsenate to be washed off more readily, despite its adhesive quality. As researchers began to test other produce, an alarming detail emerged: Unlike the apple, other fruits such as strawberries and blackberries had irregular, pitted surfaces. Coupled with the remarkable sticky properties of lead arsenate, these summer-time delicacies soaked up lead arsenate and would not let go. One study measured the amount of arsenic contained in strawberries two days after they had been sprayed and found an average of 11.5 mg of arsenic—*per* strawberry."[39] The researcher who conducted the study cautioned that "strawberries should be thoroughly scrubbed before eaten,"[40] an admonition that would be impossible to implement at commercial scale.

By 1915, authorities began seizing fruits for inspection and alarm had grown such that the U.S. Bureau of Chemistry began the most thorough study ever conducted on the safety and effects of lead arsenate on produce. Despite the exhaustive examination, it was only looking at the possibilities of acute poisoning. It didn't consider the effects of chronic accumulation, and more importantly, it didn't address the potential interaction between pesticides and pathogens. The combination of these two—metals and microbes—may have been causing far more problems than what anyone thought possible.

Chapter Twenty

Miracle of Coincidences

WITH LITTLE TO NO SCIENTIFIC STUDY ON the concept—particularly with lead arsenate—we may never know if enteroviruses are in fact given a path into the central nervous system through digestive tracts ruined by metals or pesticides. Regardless, *something* had changed that was causing more epidemics of poliomyelitis to appear each summer in cities and towns throughout the United States and other parts of the world.

It might be tempting for the layman to suggest genetic drift created a poliovirus that became more virulent sometime in the late 1800s, and this provided for a rise in paralytic infections. When viewed in light of the corpus of historical documents regarding poliomyelitis, it is clear there was a significant rise in epidemics of paralysis near the beginning of the 1900s, and a sudden mutation within the poliovirus alone cannot explain it.

For one thing, the poliovirus itself consists of three *genotypes*, all of which are capable of causing paralysis if introduced into the nervous system. For all three of them to have simultaneously mutated—and for all of them to have mutated in the same way to become *more* virulent—is a coincidence unlikely to have happened.

Even if this miraculous event were to have occurred, other enteroviruses such as coxsackievirus and echovirus would need to have mutated in such a way they could also cause paralysis more readily than they were previously capable of. While this additional happenstance may appear unlikely, the sudden appearance of paralytic afflictions amongst an assortment of animal species around this same time period—due to a variety of bacterial infections—makes the search for a genetic cause to epidemic poliomyelitis seem unlikely.

Many have suggested that improvements in sanitation caused the rise in paralytic polio. It has been proposed that advances in water quality and sewage systems created a reservoir of children that did not gain natural immunity to the poliovirus infection at a young age—as had happened in previous generations. This may seem to make sense on the surface, but does not stand up to even a trivial amount of scrutiny. The illness was called *infantile paralysis* for an obvious reason—infants were targeted time and again, as were children. It is unclear how improvements to sanitation could simultaneously prevent children from exposure *and* target them more frequently than anyone else.

Most of the outbreaks happened in rural countrysides, where the spraying of pesticides was rife. These areas were often served by well-built outhouses purposefully located far away from water supplies. They were stable locales and under no pressure from overflowing populations. Although they were not immune to the potential for enterovirus infections, nothing about their rustic living conditions would have changed significantly during that time that might have triggered epidemics of poliomyelitis. Even today—over a hundred years later—many of these rural locations still have no connections to public facilities but use well water and septic systems.

An argument could be made that the decline in breast-fed babies may have lowered their passive immunity to many of these enteroviruses. Breast milk can provide babies antibodies that can protect—or at least minimize the harm—from many common infections, depending on the mother's immunological health. Around this time period, feeding infants cow's milk or scientifically-designed formula became very popular, possibly due to the medicinal metals and ingested pesticides many women were no doubt passing on to their children.

While this hypothesis does support the fact that many of the victims were infants, Caverly documented the diet of many of the children who were stricken in Vermont and those who were breast-fed often numbered just as many as those who were not. And it still doesn't explain how so many previously innocuous microbes were gaining entry into the spinal cords to cause paralysis. Most children wouldn't be fortunate enough (or unfortunate enough) to be exposed to every enterovirus while under the protection of antibodies from their mother's milk. They would develop their own immunity after natural infections later on in their life, as teens or possibly adults. Although certainly unpleasant, these infections were not associated with paralysis until isolated cases began to appear.

It's clear that something had been altered in the late 1800s that was causing an increasing number of people—most often children—to become paralyzed. This was not an artificial spike in cases due to the improved recognition of a newly designated disease, but an unambiguous increase that had emerged from seemingly nowhere to dominate much of medical research in the early 1900s.

The one thing that had been introduced into the specific areas that began suffering *en masse* was arsenic-based pesticide. The medicinal metals of the 1800s were certainly capable of causing problems, and their administration was probably linked to isolated cases of paralysis that were sprinkled throughout that century. But as pesticides began to be applied with reckless abandon and were inadvertently ingested by nearly every living thing—adults, children, infants, not to mention animals, insects, even fish—the number of creatures that were stricken with poliomyelitis would skyrocket.

Although the 1894 Vermont epidemic was the first poliomyelitis outbreak in the United States, a few others had already occurred in rural areas of Sweden—the birthplace of lead arsenate's close cousin, Paris green. The fact that the only two countries in the late 1800s experiencing epidemics of poliomyelitis were both heavily employing native-born pesticides suggests that perhaps a rogue enterovirus was not the problem.

* * *

As World War I broke out in Europe in 1914, and America—still happily united after the scare of the Civil War—labored to keep itself out of conflict, the poliomyelitis which had sporadically appeared in epidemics across the country would become worse. Scientists were convinced they had their mark—the poliovirus—and although they would not even be able to see the virus for over another thirty years, they were beginning the seemingly impossible task of developing a protective serum, or quite possibly a vaccine against its attack.

The help could not come soon enough, for in just two years time, poliomyelitis would leave the expanse of rural America and target New York City, resulting in the deadliest epidemic the country would ever experience.

Chapter Twenty-One

Baby Week

THE EVENTS OF THE YEAR 1916 MIGHT symbolize, in retrospect, the quintessential American experience as much as nearly any year before or after. The Chicago Cubs beat the Cincinnati Reds 7-6 in their first game at Weeghman Park—later to become Wrigley Field. The Boy Scouts, the PGA, and the National Park Service were formed. An Atlanta based company began manufacturing a distinctive, contoured bottle to sell its popular drink, Coca-Cola, to discourage the numerous imposters stealing their sales. Despite the loss of over a thousand civilians on the passenger ship Lusitania—sunk a year earlier by the torpedo from a German U-boat—Woodrow Wilson was still working tirelessly to keep the United States from entering into the first World War.

In New York City, elevated trains ran down the middle of streets, passing by the Hippodrome, a performance theatre that could seat over 5,000 and regularly featured dancing elephants and horses that could dive into an enormous water tank. Many could not afford entry but lived amongst the filth of tenement housing—hastily converted buildings that stuffed far too many people in far too little space. Light was scant, fresh air was negligible, and it was not uncommon for a group of people to identify their home by a chalk outline drawn on the floor amidst several other family's rectangles. In addition to poor medical care, appalling sanitation made for deadly living conditions. Tuberculosis and diarrhea killed thousands every year, far more than measles, whooping cough, and smallpox.

Steps were being taken to improve things. The city's Board of Health met and decided to ban cyanide fumigation, a pesticide practice evidently popular at the time. Its recent "Spitting Crusade" had netted 1,740 arrests and $2,549 in fines.[41] A physical exam was conducted on 3,004 city employees, and the most common problem for women behind overweight (285) and underweight (245) was low blood pressure (235).[42] Children were sent to places like Goodhue and Holiday Farm to gain weight because they had been refused employment for being too skinny. A special club for "nervous" children was created to help them deal with a particularly annoying habit—the biting of their fingernails.

The first week of May had been designated as "Baby Week" by the mayor. Eight-hundred movie theaters promoted the campaign and 4,000 posters plastered on subways, buses, and trains announced the purpose of the drive: "Better Parents!

Better Babies! Better City!" Although New York's mortality rate was lower than the other big cities of America—Boston, Philadelphia, Chicago, and Baltimore—almost one in ten babies born would die before they reached one year old.

Mothers were taking their infants to milk stations located across the city—not to receive free bottles of pasteurized cow's milk, but to have them examined by nurses and doctors manning the kiosks in hopes their child would be selected as "the best baby in all Greater New York."[43] Many were turned away in sorrow as they were told their precious child was perhaps not as precious as they had thought.

At last, on Friday, the 3,000 infants submitted for consideration had been winnowed down to the final pair, and a team of doctors began the arduous task of determining who was the better baby—8-month-old John Ryan of 425 East 166th Street, or 19-month-old Anna Hennessy of 570 Eighty-fifth Street, Brooklyn:

> *The doctors first examined the babies' records, and then examined the babies. The mothers stood by, their hearts hardly beating. Which of them would be the mother of the champion baby of the city? Then little Anna Hennessy began to cry a little, and the doctors decided that John Ryan possessed steadier nerves and better self-control, and forthwith he was awarded the prize.*
>
> *John Ryan's father is James Ryan, 40 years old and an electrician in a large theatre. There is no prouder father today in New York City. The baby's mother, Jennie Ryan, 31 years old, would not part with the gold cup which her baby won if she did not have a cent to her name.*[44]

The Baby Week campaign had been a huge success, and though certain parts of the city were still mired in squalor, the lectures and pamphlets provided to mothers in the previous days were hoped to improve the dreadful numbers of children dying young. On Sunday—Baby Sunday—sermons were delivered from pulpits across the city emphasizing how to properly care for infants. A prayer—written specifically for that special day —was read out loud by every congregation:

> *O, God, since Thou hast laid the little children into our arms in utter helplessness, with no protection save our love, we pray that the sweet appeal of their baby hands may not be in vain. Let no innocent life in our city be quenched again in useless pain through our ignorance and sin. May we who are mothers or fathers seek eagerly to join wisdom to our love, lest love itself be deadly when unguided by knowledge. Bless the doctors and nurses, and all the friends of men, who are giving of their skill and devotion to the care of our children...*
>
> *Forgive us, our Father, for the heartlessness of the past. Grant us great tenderness for all babes who suffer, and a growing sense of the divine mystery that is brooding in the soul of every child. Amen.*[45]

The sentiment of that prayer would soon take on profound significance. Two days later, a case of infantile paralysis would appear in little Anna Hennessy's Brooklyn neighborhood. Within a month, the entire city of New York—and eventually many states beyond—would be engulfed in the deadliest epidemic of poliomyelitis the country would ever experience.

Chapter Twenty-Two

The Bad Beginning

WITH SUMMER STILL MORE THAN A MONTH away, the cases of infantile paralysis that began to surface in Brooklyn, New York, drew little attention from Haven Emerson, the city's Health Commissioner. Previous years had seen as many as 30 or 40 cases per month, so the number of children suffering—apparently less than ten—didn't set off any alarms. Diarrhea and tuberculosis were constant threats, and many of the city's milk supplier's inability to keep their products refrigerated only made things worse. As a result, Emerson spent considerable time promoting better sanitation throughout the city in an effort to arrest the spread of disease.

Like many cities, poliomyelitis had only recently become a

reportable illness. Special classes would need to be held in order to train doctors to recognize its symptoms—necessary because most had never seen it before. Infantile paralysis had been for the most part a problem in the rural country, and its spread did not follow any understandable routes. It might infect a child living in complete isolation from the outside world, sparing eight other brothers and sisters. It might infect two families whose children attended the same school but spare even the most sickly classmates. There was little that made sense about who or why certain people would be stricken down with paralysis.

As more cases began to come to light, it was clear that Brooklyn was suffering a peculiar epidemic of poliomyelitis. It was not skipping towns in the scattershot way it had done in the past—it was radiating outwards from the area of the initial outbreak.

By the 7th of June, Haven Emerson began to receive reports that more cases were beginning to appear. A curious detail accompanied the epidemiologist's account: the victims were infants, predominantly boys, as had happened in the past, but the infections seemed to target Italian children—the immigrants living amongst the muck and grime of Brooklyn. Nurses manning the milk stations began to see concerned mothers bringing their infants in to be looked at. It was clear something was wrong—their babies' arms were hanging limp by their sides, their legs completely motionless.

Another disturbing trait began to emerge—this poliomyelitis was especially deadly. Although paralysis would typically start in the baby's legs, slowly ascending the spinal column towards their arms, this outbreak could sufficiently paralyze their breathing muscles and asphyxiate them within a day. Amidst the horrors of cholera, typhoid fever, or tuberculosis—diseases that any new mother had to worry about —nothing killed as fast as what these terrified parents were seeing.

Before the end of the month, the outbreak had spread beyond Brooklyn into Manhattan, and daily accounts began to appear in local newspapers. On June 30th, it was announced that there had been 255 cases so far. Forty-nine new cases had been reported in a single day. Eleven children had died in Brooklyn, and one in Manhattan.

With the worst of summer still weeks away, Haven Emerson called a special meeting to coordinate with other Health Departments' activities in an attempt to stop the growth of the disease.

> *We believe that application of well organized sanitary measures will limit this outbreak. The Health Department cannot possibly carry out all measures necessary unless the people do their part and promptly report every case even remotely suspicious. Reports from janitors, neighbors, visiting nurses, as well as physicians will be welcomed. No names of persons making them are necessary. Our chief reliance must lie in complete and quick isolation of patients for not less than eight weeks, and on perfect cleanliness of the patient's surroundings.*[46]

A few health officials of the city made it clear there was no preventive or cure for the disease. Panic set in, and vendors began trolling the streets with hastily-made concoctions promising aid. A man was convicted for selling bags of cedar wood shavings perfumed with naphthalene as a "protector" against infantile paralysis. Another was jailed for 30 days for selling a combination of malt extract and salicylic acid as a cure.

While the World War had spared most Americans from physical duress, the outbreak of poliomyelitis in New York City was beginning to affect everyone. Seventy-five had died, all but two of them under ten years old. The hapless New York mayor's attempt at lifting the spirits of concerned parents and physicians said everything about the dire straits they found themselves in:

> *Those who could help in the war against infantile paralysis by refraining from doing things, yesterday to a large extent refrained, and those who could help by going out and doing things, to a large extent went out and did.*[47]

As the first week of summer drew to a close, it was clear to all—something different was happening. Gone were the small, rural outbreaks that had peppered the American countryside for the past twenty years. Poliomyelitis had struck the heart of the United States, and the world would notice. It was still preying on the young, particularly those who seemed the most strong and robust, but was far more lethal than anyone had ever seen before. In previous epidemics, five percent of those infected might die. So far, this was proving to be at least four times that deadly. Most alarmingly, its spread was different—it wasn't skipping towns, bouncing around randomly. It had unfurled outward from Brooklyn—evenly and fast.

Chapter Twenty-Three

Rockefeller

Another meeting, lead by the Rockefeller Institute's polio expert, Simon Flexner, was held at their headquarters in Manhattan the next day. Because the nasal washings of those suffering from poliomyelitis had sometimes produced positive results for what they assumed was the poliovirus, scientists were certain the illness was being spread through the air—if not by mosquitoes or house flies, then by coughing or sneezing. As a result, parents were warned to keep their children away from movie theaters, churches, and any gatherings of large groups of people—particularly those being held indoors.

Under the authority of Flexner, the Rockefeller Institute had taken the lead in trying to understand the nature of how the poliovirus was spreading, how it was paralyzing, and most importantly, how a preventative serum or vaccine might be developed for it. Because of the strange, unpredictable patterns in which poliomyelitis seemed to infect, discovering the mode of transmission was an important step in unlocking the mysteries of the new disease.

A few researchers appeared to have been able to transmit the poliovirus using horse flies, but others were unable to replicate their results. Scientists at the Rockefeller Institute were actively experimenting with mosquitoes in an attempt to see if they were capable of conveying the virus from one monkey to another. In fact, their efforts in spreading the poliovirus via mosquito bites would take on an ominous tone that summer as the laboratory in which they were conducting their tests was less than a mile from the epicenter of the outbreak. This coincidence has not gone unnoticed by modern historians and has been suggested as perhaps a reason for its peculiar nature. An additional quirk regarding their poliovirus research adds a bit more plausibility.

Although it was discovered that Rhesus monkeys could be infected with the poliovirus and might become paralyzed under the right conditions, it usually required an injection of the virus directly into their brain or nervous system for this to happen. This route of infection was decidedly unnatural, however. Infants were being paralyzed all over New York City—ostensibly by the poliovirus—yet they weren't being injected directly into their brain or spinal cord. They were being exposed to the enterovirus through some other way—an insect bite, a sneeze or cough, human contact—anything besides a cerebral injection.

As research regarding poliomyelitis proceeded, scientists realized they would never be able to truly understand how the poliovirus was paralyzing infants if they weren't able to study infections under more natural circumstances. A monkey could only be used once for this experiment, and as their cost was very high, scientists were reluctant to infect their tests animals in any way that wouldn't produce the desired result. They had to figure out a way to infect their test subjects more readily without resorting to nervous system injections of the virus.

A few scientists at the Rockefeller Institute had begun trying to produce a more virulent strain of the poliovirus. As a virus is passaged through multiple hosts, it will often lose its strength over time. This is how some vaccines are made—the offending virus is purposefully cycled, generation after generation, through growth medium in a way that simulates decades of attenuation. Ideally, the virus can be captured at just the right point in such a way that it will produce a strong immune response from the host in which it's introduced, but not so much that it will harm.

Maintaining this ideal balance of virulence versus the potential for harm through the millions of growth cycles it takes to produce commercial vaccines can be more art than science. Sometimes cycling a virus doesn't produce an attenuated version, but instead makes for a more virulent one—a virus that is capable of increased damage, rather than less. This is specifically what the researchers at the Rockefeller Institute hoped for as they began experimenting with the poliovirus. They were purposefully trying to create a more virulent strain in order that their expensive test monkeys might be more readily paralyzed by simply ingesting the virus.

The Rockefeller scientists were successful with their efforts, at least partially. They were able to create a dangerous strain of the poliovirus—a strain that evidently multiplied extremely aggressively within neuronal cells. Monkeys were much more likely to become paralyzed from this special type of poliovirus they had been able to create. These experiments—with an extremely dangerous poliovirus strain alongside the mosquito transmission studies—were being run that very year in a laboratory a mile up the East River from the nucleus of the most deadly poliomyelitis outbreak in history.

It would seem the accidental release of an especially vicious poliovirus so close to Brooklyn might offer an explanation as to what was causing the particularly deadly epidemic of poliomyelitis. Perhaps the thousands of mosquitoes they were testing transmission with escaped or were inadvertently released into the sewage system and *were* able to spread the new poliovirus in such a way that had previously been impossible.

Although the experiments with mosquitoes and mutant poliovirus strains so close in time and proximity to the outbreak may seem like more than just coincidence, closer inspection suggests they may not be related at all. The bulk of mosquito experiments actually happened later in the year, after the summer was over. The studies involved jars of mosquitoes small enough to sit comfortably on laboratory counters—quantities of insects so few they would be unlikely to make the mile journey to Brooklyn without causing a disturbance along the way. Researchers have since been unable to promote the transmission of the poliovirus through mosquitoes, so it would appear the flying creatures at Rockefeller Institute might not be involved.

It is tempting to suppose the inadvertent release of the special strain of poliovirus produced at the lab that year might explain the reason poliomyelitis was so deadly. As it turns out, the virus did have an increased affinity for the nervous system but had a *decreased* affinity for replicating anywhere else—it was nearly impossible to cultivate outside of the nervous system. The breathtaking pattern of growth seen in New York and beyond resembled something with a remarkable ability to spread. Even if the virus was more *neurotropic*, it still didn't explain how it got into the nervous system in the first place—it was a virus more deadly within the nervous system, but if anything, had *less* ability to get there in the first place.

Furthermore, scientists quickly discovered that over multiple generations, the virus would revert back to the tame version of its previous self—causing no more harm than a natural variant. Maintaining the virulent type of the virus was difficult, and they eventually abandoned its development. While the Rockefeller strain of the poliovirus may have initially caused an increase in the mortality of those it infected, its deadliness should have decreased quickly over time. Unfortunately, that is not what would happen in New York.

Chapter Twenty-Four

July, 1916

By July 4th, Haven Emerson's efforts to control the outbreak had become dramatic. The day before, 72 new cases of infantile paralysis occurred, and twenty-three had died. Independence Day celebrations were cancelled throughout the city, and children under 16 were banned from local movie theaters. Even the Nickelodeons and free, open-air screenings for children were scrapped. The Society for the Prevention of Cruelty to Animals increased its efforts to round up stray dogs and cats, increasing the number of creatures destroyed from 300 to 450 every day.

Many of the city health officers and other physicians spent their holiday scouring apartment buildings and playgrounds for children showing any signs of being sick, often finding what they took as foreboding signs—uncovered trash cans, litter in the hallways, or windows with no protective screens. Volunteers from two insurance companies and the Department of Health distributed 500,000 leaflets around the city to warn those who were unaware:

> *INFANTILE PARALYSIS (POLIOMYELITIS)*
>
> *Infantile paralysis is very prevalent in this part of the city. Keep your children out of the street as much as possible, and be sure to keep them out of the houses on which the Department of Health has put a sign.*
>
> *The daily paper will tell you in what house the disease is. This is the disease which babies and young children get; many of them die, and many who do not, become paralyzed for life. Do not let your children go to parties, picnics, or outings.*

Proposals were floated to keep all children under the age of sixteen housebound for two weeks, but the ensuing illness from other diseases was thought likely to offset any reduction in poliomyelitis. A social worker who had been canvassing apartments in search of undiscovered infantile paralysis wrote a letter of concern to the head of the Volunteer Hospital at which she was employed:

> *My Dear Miss Sand: Conditions are dreadful here this year. We cannot send any of our poor children away, and that means they must stay in the hot, dirty houses in the hot, dirty streets without a change of any kind. I fear there will be as many deaths from that as from the "disease," as it is called by the poor. The mothers are so afraid that most of them will not even let the*

> *children enter the streets, and some will not even have a window open. In one house I went into the only window was not only shut, but the cracks were stuffed with rags so that the "disease" could not come in. You can imagine what the dark, dirty room was like: the babies had no clothes on, and were so hot they looked as if they had been dipped in oil, and the flies were sticking all over them. I had to tell the mother I would get the Board of Health after her to make her open the window, and now if any of the children do get infantile paralysis she will feel that I killed them. I do not wonder they are afraid. I went to see one family about 4 P.M. Friday. The baby was not well and the doctor was coming. When I returned Monday morning there were three little hearses before the door; all her children had been swept away in that short time. The mothers are hiding their children rather than give them up, so now it is said the plague is on the wane; but it is really worse than admitted.*[48]

If a child was suspected to be ill, the officials would take them to a hospital, with police force if necessary, unless the parents could convince them they would abide by their strict sanitation and quarantine measures—eight weeks in an isolated room within their apartment. If they were allowed to remain at home, red and white placards would be placed outside their building, beside their apartment door, and a third—inside the residence beside the sick room door—to announce they were under quarantine and that no one outside the immediate family besides the direct caretaker was to enter. The warning would stay beyond the quarantine until the room the child lived in was completely disinfected, including new wall paper—a curious repair request considering its troubled association with Paris green dyes.

For the parents who didn't have a separate room for

isolation, their sick child would be taken from them by ambulance to one of several hospital wards throughout the city. The isolation and quarantine rules at the hospital reflected the grave situation New York found itself in: Parents were not allowed to visit, for any reason. Some wards had ground-level windows through which parents could observe their children, but most were unable to even see them and were limited to verbal updates from a nurse. Toys, books, or articles of clothing from home—anything that might have offered comfort to the poor children—were not allowed. If they survived their hospital stay, everything that had been donated to them—even library books—were burned.

Besides less filth, fewer flies, and the draft a few open windows provided, hospitals could offer little improvement over a dirty mattress in a chalk square in the middle of a Brooklyn tenement floor. Poliomyelitis was unlike anything else they treated, specifically because the children appeared to be healthy. Other than the initial fever and malaise which often signaled the onset of an infection, paralysis was the only symptom that remained. They were not lethargic, sleepy, or otherwise incapacitated—their exuberant spirit often a more common symptom than gloomy despair. Indeed the strongest, most healthy children seemed more likely to be struck down—an occurrence which made infantile paralysis all the more cruel.

Doctors and nurses were left with few options to treat them. Rest, fresh air, and quiet were provided. Massage was offered for patients who could stand it, and those who were suffering from constipation due to their bowels being paralyzed were given mercury-containing calomel—sometimes in massive doses. For children with severe paralysis, their limbs or trunks were bound up tightly in plaster or braces in a futile—and often excruciating—attempt to prevent their atrophying muscles from warping their bones. Most alarmingly, there was nothing doctors could do to slow the ascent of poliomyelitis up the spinal cord towards the lungs.

On July 15th, a large group of physicians and health officials met at the Rockefeller Institute to discuss what could be done about the growing outbreak. They were mesmerized by the presentation from a prominent researcher and physician who lived in Harlem. Dr. S.J. Meltzer had experienced success in treating monkeys sick with poliomyelitis by injecting adrenaline directly into their spinal cords.

> *Animals which were paralyzed and moribund at the time of the injection were seen several hours later eating bananas which they held themselves. The paralytic conditions were strikingly improved and the life of the animals was prolonged in some cases for several days. The animals finally died, but in this series of Dr. Clark's experiments, all animals received reliably fatal doses of the virus.*[49]

Emboldened by the results—and desperate to help—he made a recommendation to the physicians in attendance that they "inject adrenaline intraspinally in every case of infantile paralysis."[50] Although his proposal would be taken to heart by many doctors throughout the city, Health Commissioner Haven Emerson made it clear excitement over the experimental treatment may have been premature, saying in his typically understated way, "I do not wish to detract from what Dr.

Meltzer has done, but his paper was made disproportionately prominent in the newspaper reports of Thursday night's discussion."[51]

Before Dr. Meltzer finished speaking, he brought up one last suggestion based on some research he had been doing for several years. He described an apparatus he had developed—a bellows of some sort—which could be used to administer artificial respiration "as soon as the patient shows a degree of unconsciousness and respiratory insufficiency."[52]

His allotted time had expired, and Meltzer ended his presentation without any further explanation as to how the device worked or might be used on children. It did not matter —the adrenaline research had captured everyone's attention and physicians left the meeting euphoric with the hope they could finally begin to help.

Chapter Twenty-Five

August, 1916

By the end of July, the outbreak of infantile paralysis had become much worse than anyone could have imagined. Fifty-five people had died in a single day—the highest number yet recorded. 159 new cases had been reported—also one of the highest number of cases up to that point. The dreaded disease had spread to nearby Newark, New Jersey, and several other neighboring states had begun to see their numbers shoot up dramatically.

Draconian measures were being put into place—not only within the city, but outside it. During July, parents who could afford to were putting their children on trains and sending them far away, to any friend or relative who would take them.

In a typical summer, many of the poorest children were normally taken out of the city for "Fresh Air" trips to nearby lakes or camps, but by the time August came, they would find it very difficult to get out of the city. The fresh air trips for the poor were cancelled. Many children who left by rail in search of safety were not allowed off the train if they weren't carrying a certificate of clean health. Most summer camps were already full of poliomyelitis refugees and would not chance sparking their own epidemic by allowing anyone else to enter. Even food deliveries were dropped off far away from the children and picked up by employees who were known to be uninfected.

For those that were forced to stay, the misery of quarantine and isolation was compounded by the unbearable heat of midsummer. Normally, families would leave their stifling apartments at night and sleep on bridges or as close to the water as they could safely get. Now, they were forced to stay inside their apartments, and children who were sick couldn't even leave during the day.

* * *

With no way to escape the high temperatures, many of the public baths around the city were swarmed with both children and adults. These large buildings began as floating pool houses with changing rooms on various bodies of water but were eventually constructed as permanent buildings throughout neighborhoods in an attempt to give the poor a chance to clean themselves. While this may seem like an affront to the less-fortunate, in 1893 only 2% of families in New York City had a bathroom within their house or tenement. By 1916, the number was only slightly better.

Even so, bathrooms were not thought of as an opportunity to get clean. A photograph from that era, entitled "The Only Bathtub on the Block," depicts what some tenement dwellers thought of this hygienic contrivance—it was hanging outside a window, presumably to make room for more storage or sleeping in their cramped living quarters. Cultural moires of the time did not encourage frequent bathing, and as such, hygiene obsessed health officials had the foresight to secure funding to erect two and three-story public baths.

Although their most popular feature were the large indoor pools, they were designed for people to bathe and contained many private stalls with tile floors, toilets, and what must have been in wintertime the absolute revelation of a hot shower. Most designs provided for nearly twice as many male "rain baths" as female, and buildings that were completely gender segregated were often open only one or two days a week for females. Swimming was seen by many as unfit recreation for women and girls, partly due to the lack of proper attire for females. Males could strip down to their underwear and call it a swimsuit while women were forced to rent a fifteen-pound wool garment.

Nevertheless, a July letter to the editor from a concerned citizen gave clear indication to how popular these baths had become:

To the Editor of the New York Times:

The other day I stood for more than three hours in the line waiting to get into the public bath at Coney Island.

Why shouldn't our city build more public baths? They would be

highly appreciated by citizens.
Harry Hellerman,
Brooklyn, July 9, 1916.[53]

Pictures of public baths from that era show hundreds of boys, stacked up on top of each other behind railings around the pool's edge, waiting for their chance to plunge into the cool drink. Knowing that most enteroviruses can be spread through contaminated water makes one wonder if whatever was causing the soaring poliomyelitis that summer was being given a helping-hand by public swimming pools, teeming with possibly both children *and* microbes. The fact that boys were targeted with paralysis more frequently than girls makes this hypothesis all the more intriguing.

Health officials would not have strongly suspected contaminated swimming pools as a possible source of infection and, indeed, were more fearful of dust than water. Dust and dirt were seen as mortal enemies of good sanitation—just as capable of disease transmission as flies or mosquitoes—and had been positioned for years as the cause of much infantile suffering. As a result, mothers focused more of their cleaning on grime and were blissfully unaware of the thousands of microbes staining their sinks from washing cloth diapers or coating the floors where trash and refuse had piled up for days.

This battle against dust was not the providence of women alone and was taken on in epic fashion by the city's Street Cleaning Department, whose leader promised "180 gangs of men working day and night if the Department of Water Supply could furnish 4,000,000 gallons of water daily."[54] Police pitched in to help, diligently looking for and fining anyone they caught not using covered trash containers.

Besides removing the tons of refuse that was carelessly tossed into streets and sidewalks every day, the street cleaning department was determined to minimize the amount of harmful dust that would otherwise accumulate. Announcements were made to assure the public that dirt would not be a contributing factor in the spread of infantile paralysis that summer.

> *In Brooklyn, where the epidemic has been most severe, the number of hose gangs employed in night flushing will be increased from fifteen to forty in the affected areas. Night work will be increased by 50 per cent.*[55]

Knowing the kind of filth that was being flushed into drainage systems in New York every day would give anyone pause as to what kind of secondary health effects it might have had. A prominent Swedish poliomyelitis researcher, who had seen his fair share of epidemic polio in his home country, voiced serious concerns about the street flushing:

> *...it was his belief that the rapid spread of the disease in New York was due to the way in which the streets were cleaned—watered and swept first, after which the garbage was hauled over them, and then children allowed to play in them. Dr. Hoving thought garbage should be hauled in first, and then the streets cleaned. He said all large European cities had learned the lesson New York had not.*[56]

Although the combination of heat, crowded public bathing, and aggressive street flushing may have inadvertently been working against ending the epidemic, it wasn't a drastically different sequence of events than had occurred any other summer. Yet despite the most aggressive efforts at isolation and quarantine the country ever experienced, the disease had thundered past any line of defense they could muster.

Their inability to stop the spread of infantile paralysis was made all the more curious because of areas which were spared: orphanages and children's homes. These public run facilities may have promoted better sanitation and hygiene than other areas of the city, but in light of the apparent futility of public health efforts without, it was truly remarkable when a place which 2,000 children called home did not come down with a single case. Even more curious was the situation at Barren Island:

> *There were 350 children, under 16 years of age, on Barren Island in Jamaica Bay, Borough of Brooklyn. To this Island all the city garbage and offal is taken for reduction in the large rendering plants. Flies and mosquitoes are abundant. Rats are numerous. There is no public water supply and there are many shallow surface water wells. There is no sewage system. There are few, if any, cellars. There is no garbage collection. There are no public highways. The population of about 1,300 people represents the lower grade of unskilled labor, Poles, Italians and Negroes predominating. The standard of living is low. No cases of poliomyelitis developed on Barren Island.*[57]

It is bizarre that improvements in sanitation appeared to offer little protection to most of New York, while children living within the confines of publicly-run children's homes were saved. The 350 children living amongst the squalor of Barren

Island were similarly protected, as were the 80 or 90 children living on Governor's Island, a nearby military post.

The segregation offered by the orphanages—along with those living in seclusion on islands and military bases—may have been enough of a firewall to keep the disease at bay. But to confound a possible explanation, in rural areas, isolation seemed to offer no protection against the disease. Stories abounded of infantile paralysis striking children on farms that drank from deep well water, were a mile away from their nearest neighbor, and hadn't seen a visitor for weeks.

It is important to recall that poliomyelitis was known to have multiple causes. The rural cases of poliomyelitis were likely the same source as Rutland, Vermont's 1894 epidemic—arsenic poisoning from the new pesticides heavily applied to nearly everything they ate. It's probable that an enterovirus such as the poliovirus occasionally *did* cross the path of a child whose guts were wrecked from ingesting lead arsenate or medicinal metals administered to them for an unrelated illness, an occurrence which might explain the rare case where more than one child from the same family was struck.

Within the city, many of the thousands of people coming down with infantile paralysis were no doubt being poisoned by these same metals. But something else was going on—this epidemic clearly had a proclivity for transmission that had never been seen before. Lead arsenate poisoning alone could not explain the way the outbreak had started in Brooklyn and radiated outwardly, nor could the fecal-oral transmission route of a trivial enterovirus which had infected millions of people for hundreds of years with apparently little harm.

As August drew to a close, any dip in the number of new

cases or deaths was trumpeted by all as the long-awaited harbinger of the end. New records were still being broken across the state of New York, but within the city it appeared that perhaps the worst was behind them. Almost eight-thousand — mostly children—had been stricken with the disease. Nearly 2,000 were dead. Autumn could not come fast enough for Haven Emerson and the exhausted physicians, nurses, health officials, police, street cleaning crews, and everyone else in New York City battling to save the lives of their precious children.

At the Rockefeller Institute, scientists continued their attempts to understand how the recently discovered poliovirus was spreading and reaching the heavily defended central nervous system. Another scientist following the outbreak closely made an intriguing discovery that challenged everything those at the Rockefeller laboratories were studying. According to the experiments he was conducting, the 1916 outbreak was not caused by a virus at all, but a very odd bacteria—a special type of microbe no one had ever seen before.

Chapter Twenty-Six

Rosenow

THE POLIOMYELITIS OUTBREAK OF 1916 WAS UNLIKE anything the world had ever seen. It was more deadly, it infected more readily, and its spread took on different characteristics than anything before or since. Enterovirus infections alone couldn't explain the paralysis experienced by so many that summer. More bewildering—the path of destruction resembled nothing like the way the fecal-oral transmission route of an enterovirus might spread.

At the time, the explanation of how other diseases spread began to fall into place. It had been revealed that mosquitoes could spread disease amongst humans, as could certain ticks. New microbes were being discovered left and right, and for scientists with their powerful microscopes, it was truly an age of discovery. As they sought to understand the cause of various diseases, a set of criteria known as Koch's postulates were created to determine whether a particular bacteria was the true cause of illness. The postulates stated that Germ X must be found in all organisms suffering from Disease X, but not in healthy organisms. Germ X should be isolated from someone suffering from Disease X and introduced into a healthy organism, where it should cause them to also develop Disease X. Finally, Germ X must be recovered from *that* recently infected organism.

Over time, these postulates lost their appeal as it was realized they had limited utility, but in the early 1900s, the search for the cause of poliomyelitis was shaped by vigorous adherence to these criteria. Because of this, they assumed there was a *single* microbe which caused poliomyelitis. They assumed that single microbe should never be found in healthy subjects. And finally, it meant they assumed this particular microbe should always cause paralysis if introduced into a healthy subject. In retrospect, we know there were several—if not many—causes of poliomyelitis, and consequently the narrow search specified by Koch's postulates should have ended in vain.

While some scientists were trying to isolate the virus they believed to be causing poliomyelitis, others were convinced it was actually caused by a bacteria. One such scientist was named Edward Rosenow, thought to be one of the most brilliant scientists alive. He was head of experimental bacteriology at the Mayo Foundation and his inventions, such as the Rosenow Sterile Air Chamber, were being used by scientists around the world to ensure microbes did not contaminate their experiments.

Rosenow was able to get tissue samples directly from victims of the 1916 New York epidemic and was surprised to routinely find a form of the *streptococcus* bacteria. He was also able to consistently cause poliomyelitis by injecting this bacteria in various research animals. Finally, he was able to retrieve the bacteria from the animals once they had died. Being an extremely thorough researcher, Rosenow conducted these studies on over 2,000 experimental animals and was convinced he had found the cause of poliomyelitis, even by Koch's strict criteria for causality.

There was a problem, however. Others could not always replicate his results. A few scientists who followed his directions precisely were able to, but many were confused by some of the idiosyncrasies of his laboratory techniques. Rosenow was describing something they had never heard of before—a new form of streptococcus bacteria that took on strange shapes and were so small they could not be seen on traditional microscopes. To add to the confusion, they could pass straight through the filters that would typically block any normal bacteria from passing.

* * *

Microbiology is not the exact science many think of it as. Peering through a microscope does not always reveal discrete microbial forms that can be easily classified within a clearly delineated taxonomy. Bacteria can change forms, often in ways that make recognition difficult. Some take on round shapes, others look like rods, while still others are curved or even tightly spiraled. Over years of trial and error, chemical solutions were created that could stain certain bacteria in order to make them more easily identifiable. Because not all bacteria would stain, this became an attribute in and of itself that could be used to help determine what someone was looking at.

Rosenow, having studied bacterial infections within the brain for many years, was keenly aware of this. He knew that bacteria could shift and slide around in ways that were difficult to detect—sometimes becoming so small they could apparently pass through their most delicate filters, an ability which led many scientists to refer to them as viruses. Nowadays, we differentiate the two because bacteria can replicate on their own, whereas viruses require a host—another living cell. This crucial difference was not understood at the time, and as such, the ability to pass through Berkeland filters was what determined if something was classified as a virus or bacteria—it was their apparent size, not their mode of reproduction.

Years later, antibiotics would exploit this characteristic of bacteria to great effect. The penicillin family of drugs work specifically by causing bacteria to lose their cell wall—a dramatic event which effectively kills them. Unfortunately, some bacteria are not bothered the least bit by this process and, in fact, can begin replicating inside other living cells—just like viruses—a process with ramifications so nocuous as to deserve its own book. Because Rosenow sensed that some of the streptococcus bacteria he had cultured from poliomyelitis victims were transforming into a "virus" state, he sought the assistance of a fellow scientist who had built a unique microscope that could see far beyond anything possible at the time.

Dr. Royal Rife, better known for an invention that could use specifically tuned radio waves to destroy certain bacteria—while leaving other cells untouched—had created an ingenious series of optical devices he called "Universal Microscopes." These complex appliances used intersecting prisms to illuminate specific wavelengths of light in such a way that strange forms of bacteria became visible in a way that other microscopes could not reveal—no matter their magnification.

Traditional microscopy and staining techniques were unable to confirm Rosenow's assertion of the relationship between the streptococcus bacteria and poliomyelitis, so with several filtrates of his streptococcus in hand, he traveled to San Diego and spent several days with Dr. Rife and his universal microscopes. Working together, they were able to visually confirm the presence of strange forms of bacteria that had never been seen before. It was a miraculous discovery as slides that appeared crystal clear under the microscope could instantly reveal moving forms of life with a twist of the prism—without a change in focus or magnification.

* * *

The tissue samples gathered from poliomyelitis victims in 1916 clearly indicated streptococcus bacteria infection. These microbes—when cultured under special techniques Rosenow had developed—could change into a different form not visible on traditional microscopes and would readily cause poliomyelitis in test animals. Even Simon Flexner, head of the Rockefeller Institute, came to a similar conclusion through years of research he'd been conducting. According to him, a special form of microbes he called "globoid bodies" was the cause of poliomyelitis. He did not have the perspective—or clarity—Rife's Universal Microscopes had provided Rosenow, but regardless, two of the world's foremost scientists had simultaneously come to the conclusion that a strange microbial form was causing poliomyelitis.

Rosenow was consistently able to create the *poliomyelitic streptococcus* by culturing the bacteria within a special growth medium. In a normal setting, it would not work, but under certain conditions, something very odd would happen to the bacterial form. Perhaps the lead arsenate that had become prevalent in the diet of so many was able to combine with a common streptococcus infection to create a similarly diabolical form of the bacteria Rosenow had so confidently attributed to poliomyelitis. It could certainly explain the explosive spread of the disease the world was witnessing that summer, in the same way an enterovirus could not. And it could also make clear why populations of isolated children seemed to avoid the illness, no matter their living conditions or water supply.

Curiously, 1916 was one of the first large poliomyelitis epidemics that did not feature paralyzed animals alongside their human counterparts. Dead animals had been piled up everywhere, but thorough checks with the veterinarians of the city determined they had not died from paralysis but had been purposefully killed in attempt to stop the disease.

Finally, the insistence of many that infantile paralysis was originating from contaminated milk supplies may have had some validity. While vendors were thoroughly checked and no apparent problems found, the cows themselves—now being drenched in "cattle dip" arsenic baths as part of routine pesticide control—were known to excrete arsenic into the milk itself. Unrefrigerated milk is a perfect bacterial growth medium and if it contained arsenic, perhaps—along with the heat of summer—it bested Rosenow's special formula and allowed for the creation of poliomyelitic streptococcus—a strange bacterial form that could pass through the smallest filters and maybe even survive the extreme heat of pasteurization. A quick look through the Health Department's records indicates they knew there were problems with milk that summer—they destroyed nearly twice as much as the year before, a foreboding omen to this decidedly cursory hypothesis.

Due to the prevailing assumption that all poliomyelitis was attributable to a single cause, and because the idiosyncrasies of bacterial shape-shifting were poorly understood, Rosenow's insistence that a strange form of streptococcus was the cause of poliomyelitis fell into the shadows. The search for a solitary virus—and not a bacteria—causing poliomyelitis would consume nearly everyone. The scientific world was unaware the stranglehold Koch's postulates had put on their research—a mistake whose reverberations are still being felt today.

* * *

As the summer of 1916 drew to a close, the cases of infantile paralysis finally began to wane. New York City's beleaguered Haven Emerson reluctantly began allowing children as young as 12 back into movie theaters, and dates were set for schools and universities to reopen. New York lost 2,448 people to poliomyelitis, with almost 9,000 others who survived to suffer a lifetime of debilitating illness. Because poliomyelitis was such a new phenomenon, many states did not consider it a reportable disease, causing official numbers to be woefully inaccurate. Regardless, across the country, it is estimated that 27,000 people were stricken with the disease, and an additional 6,000 were killed.

Infantile paralysis had existed for years in relative obscurity —the 123 people stricken in Rutland, Vermont, twenty-two years earlier were known to nearly no one. And although the nation was about to sacrifice many of its young men in an epic struggle in Europe to help end *the Great War*, most parents were more concerned about this new threat than anything the Germans could muster.

They were right to be worried. Despite the cloud of Koch's postulates which guided everything they did, scientists were reluctantly going to have to expand the list of causes of poliomyelitis.

Chapter Twenty-Seven

Rochester, 1920

THE YEAR WAS 1920, AND IT WAS summer in Rochester, New York. Every day, forty anxious children would walk with their parents into the reception area inside the Eastman Dental Hospital where—after some paperwork was signed—the children were escorted by nurses into an examination hall. Their parents would leave and would not see them again for two days. Inside, the children were "checked, numbered, cleared, bathed, examined, put into clean night clothes, bed slippers, and a blanket, and put to bed to the delights of movies and record concerts."[58] When children had trouble going to sleep, nurses would sing uplifting songs—"It's A Grand Old Flag" or "Yankee Doodle Dandy."

In the morning, the children would be ushered into a large operating suite with four sheet-covered platforms in the center of the room. One by one, they were laid on the sheet and given anesthesia. After waiting a few minutes, a doctor would open their mouth, insert a metal snare, and snip out their tonsils and adenoids. By noon, all forty children would be recuperating from surgery, back on their cots, where they would spend another restless night until the next day when they were sent home by taxis.

This procedure was repeated every day that summer for seven weeks. Almost 1,500 children in Rochester had their tonsils and adenoids removed that summer, but the facilities were clearly not big enough. There were many more on the waiting list, thousands by many accounts—children who had been directed by school nurses and doctors to have the surgery whether or not they or their parents wanted it.

So vital was this effort considered that the surgeries had been rendered for free. The patrons of the hospital who had donated time and money to ensure this accomplishment was completed were no doubt pleased with their efforts. In a hospital-published report of the results, their satisfaction was obvious:

> *The work has spelled opportunity for Rochester's children. Every child, no matter what the circumstances of its parents, had been given an opportunity to have its teeth properly cared for, to have its tonsils and adenoids removed and so to defend the chief portals of entry, the mouth and nose, against disease.*[59]

Many years earlier, George Eastman, a Rochester resident

who spent much of his time caring for his widowed mother and polio-stricken sister, had perfected the technique of preparing dry emulsion film. He would would turn his business—Eastman Kodak—into the largest photography company in the world. Like many wealthy tycoons of the era, he had given large sums of money to improve the health and welfare of the less fortunate. Eastman's focus began with dentistry—a godsend for poor children throughout Rochester—and eventually expanded its reach into medicine's emerging fascination with tonsil and adenoid removal.

Since the turn of the century, tonsils had become a constant concern to physicians. They were thought to be the seat of inflammation for many different diseases a child might experience. Others assumed that inflamed tonsils were the actual source of infection for sickness. Nearly everyone agreed that diseased tonsils caused mouth-breathing, something they considered a clear sign of mental handicap.

In an attempt to understand this phenomenon, extensive studies were conducted at different schools. Teachers would sort their students into groups of Bright, Normal, Dull, and Dullest children. After examination by visiting physicians or nurses, the Dull and Dullest groups were noted to have had the highest number of tonsil and adenoid conditions. Although the perceived association was strong, it was not a new revelation.

Inflamed tonsils and adenoids—and the mouth breathing that went along with it—were long suspected to be the cause of nearly any mental handicap. Even 2,000 years ago, Hippocrates wrote, "Open-mouthed youths are sluggards." While this association may seem implausible, recent scientific evidence may actually support it. It is now known that a particular injected metal—aluminum hydroxide—tends to gather in the lymph nodes and what are called *lymphoid tissues.* Among other problems, the ensuing inflammation causes swelling and tenderness. In an age of frequently administered metallic medicines or pesticides, it would not be unreasonable to anticipate both swollen tonsils *and* "dull" children.

Regardless of the cause, doctors told mothers that the removal of the tonsils of their "backward child" would make them bright. Medical journals reported on the incredible intellectual improvement shown by children who had tonsillectomies. Classmates ceased making fun of them, and teachers remarked at how their test scores skyrocketed. Even perceived physical shortcomings could be cured by the magic procedure, as reports would mention children growing several inches in the months following their operations. For nearly anything that ailed a developing child, physicians had a new solution—a surgery, no less, which they could charge handsomely for.

With improvements to anesthesia and medical instruments such as the tonsil guillotine, physicians and health officials flooded into schools all over the country, looking for signs of diseased or inflamed tonsils. Children who were judged to have the disorder were sent home with a consent card which notified their parents of the supposed defect their children were experiencing and the miraculous change they should expect to see after their surgery. Clinics like the one in Rochester opened to ensure no child was heartlessly allowed to suffer the effects of mouth breathing and swollen adenoids. As a result, tonsillectomies would become the most common surgery in the country for several decades.

* * *

More and more children began getting tonsillectomies, and a disturbing trend began to materialize—if someone happened to get poliomyelitis after a recent tonsillectomy, it was more often that not, a special type of paralysis called *bulbar poliomyelitis*. The more common type, *spinal poliomyelitis*, starts at the bottom of the spinal cord and affects the legs. Sometimes the lesions ascend up the cord and affect the arms—possibly even the ability to breathe. This other type of poliomyelitis seemed to originate much higher—directly within the brain stem in an area called the medulla oblongata, a part of the brain which used to be called the *bulb* due to its curious shape.

This part of the brain is important because many of the twelve cranial nerves originate from this location. Cranial nerves are different than the nerves which branch off the spinal cord and control your arms and legs. These nerves come off the brain stem itself and—among other sensory functions like seeing, hearing, and smelling—control the muscles in your head used for moving your eyes, mouth, even swallowing and speaking. A crucial cranial nerve, the 10th *vagus* nerve, is used to regulate the heart rate and breathing cycles. If someone develops poliomyelitis in this area of their brain, they might develop facial palsy, speech disorders, or difficulty eating due to their inability to swallow. If the vagus nerve develops problems, it can disrupt their heart rate or respiration, causing death.

Fortunately, this type of poliomyelitis was very rare, making up about 2% of paralytic cases, but for those who suffered its effects, it could be just as debilitating as the more common spinal paralysis. As both tonsillectomies and the epidemics of infantile paralysis became more common in the 1900s, it didn't take long for parents—and eventually physicians—to accept that the surgery seemed to predispose someone to the bulbar form.

The medical community continued their enchantment with tonsillectomies and produced research claiming that the surgery helped *avoid* the possibility of bulbar paralysis. Nevertheless, scientists already researching poliomyelitis were keen to understand this event and began experimenting on monkeys to see if they could replicate the phenomenon—removing the tonsils from their test subjects, then days later swabbing their throats with what they believed to contain poliovirus.

Results were mixed, but it was pointed out that for many children who experienced this unfortunate event, the poliovirus—known to be found in the folds of the nasopharynx—was likely already present before surgery was performed. Even future poliovirus vaccine inventor Albert Sabin performed similar tests himself, no doubt eager to see if there was a more natural—and reliable—method of paralyzing test monkeys besides injections directly into the nervous system.

Why was this association likely? Just as the intestinal infections of certain enteroviruses typically cause paralysis in a particular section of the spinal cord they are lying adjacent to, the bulb area of the brain lies less than an inch away from the tonsils. These two geographic correlations are likely not coincidences.

In the case of tonsillectomies and bulbar poliomyelitis, it's not just their proximity that causes a problem. The poliovirus, like some other enteroviruses, replicates easily within nervous tissue. The nervous system is well protected from a viral infection—usually. If there is a viral—or possibly even bacterial—infection located in the tonsils, the trauma of their removal is likely to expose nerve endings to the infecting microbes. Days, possibly weeks later, as the tissue is still healing from the surgery, the likelihood of a neurotropic virus finding its mark is greatly increased.

Once that particular virus hits the exposed nerve ending, it can easily replicate up through the nerve, possibly all the way to the origin in the medulla oblongata. As this infection progresses, the body's immune system is called into action and will race to develop enough antibodies to clear the invader. In a suppressed immune system, the infection may progress throughout the bulb, causing massive cranial nerve damage, possibly even death.

* * *

While the occurrence of tonsillectomies and bulbar poliomyelitis was not frequent enough to slow the march of surgeons and their metallic snares, eager to correct the mouth breathing and associated mental handicaps of children across the country, a new medical procedure—also being practiced on children—was beginning to cause serious concern that it might be inadvertently causing poliomyelitis.

Chapter Twenty-Eight

The Syringe

THE HUMAN BODY IS WELL PROTECTED FROM foreign microbes. The intestines form a nearly impenetrable shield to defend against anything harmful you might ingest. Millions—possibly billions—of helpful bacteria coat the lining of your gut and can usually prevent harmful germs from gaining a foothold. The mucosal lining of your nose, mouth, throat, and lungs offers similar protection—an immune system in and of itself that guards against harmful invaders.

Your skin—called the largest organ in your body—is teeming with millions of bacteria and viruses at any given time, yet suffers no ill effects from their presence. Even parasites—often in the form of worms that live in our guts—can be co-opted by the body in an effort to control an otherwise troublesome attack. It is not a perfect system, but in general, most humans go through their daily life unaware of the epic battles being waged throughout the external facing components of their immune system.

Nature has provided some creatures with the ability to overcome these defenses. Arthropods, a huge grouping of animals with exoskeletons—which includes bees, wasps, even scorpions—often have stingers with which they can pierce the skin and inject venom. Other creatures such as snakes and spiders use their fangs to puncture the dermis before depositing their poison. Parasites—which can cause diseases like malaria, yellow fever, and filariasis—can be transmitted via the saliva of a mosquito bite, a diabolical skill that ticks and fleas also possess.

Even the infections of tetanus and rabies need a helping hand. Outside the body, they are innocuous microbes that rarely harm. If a deep skin puncture occurs from the bite of an animal—or the infamous stepping on a rusty nail injury—it can push the virus or bacteria into the nervous tissue. Rust has nothing to do with it—once in contact with nervous tissue, the tetanus and rabies microbes can replicate easily and will cause very bad problems.

The poliovirus, like all of the other paralyzing pathogens, is no different. It is a relatively innocuous virus anywhere outside of the nervous system, but inside the nervous system, it can kill. As scientists struggled to understand why children were being stricken with a new form of paralysis that had been so infrequent, a new source of poliomyelitis for children appeared which no one had expected—the syringe.

* * *

Throughout the late 1800s, physicians began looking for ways to deliver effective doses of their metallic medicines without destroying the teeth and guts of their patients in the process. Although morphine was one of the earliest medical injections, mercury became a popular shot for treating syphilis. Due to the inherent pain and danger of poorly fabricated needles, this procedure was not a common occurrence.

As the 1900s arrived, physicians began experimenting with serums and anti-toxins for the diphtheria and tetanus bacteria. By taking the blood from horses infected with these diseases, it was suspected they could administer the plasma into the uninfected—or recently infected—and grant them protection or recovery from the illness. There was no way to get this protective serum into the human body other than injecting it directly.

While the smallpox vaccine had existed for a hundred years, it was less of an injection and more of a scrape. A bifurcated needle was used to scratch the skin and administer the inoculum subcutaneously. The diphtheria and tetanus serums were different. They were injections—deep skin punctures.

The introduction of horse blood into humans was not without problems. It heralded the introduction of two new medical concepts—*allergy* and *anaphylaxis*. As improvements were made to the sterilization of horse blood, the chances of developing rashes, joint pain, and shock after these injections fell. But another disturbing phenomenon began to surface—

poliomyelitis, following vaccination.

First noticed in 1907, reports began to appear of people developing paralysis directly after their injections. It wasn't spinal poliomyelitis, where their legs or arms were affected, and it wasn't bulbar poliomyelitis, where their cranial nerves developed problems. It was a localized paralysis that began directly at the injection site and could occasionally travel all the way into the brain or spinal cord—ending with death.

Some of it was attributed to the contamination of the shot itself. Because vaccines are often cultured in animal tissue, the chance of rogue viruses or bacteria corrupting an injection are very high. At the time, there were few safeguards in place to prevent this, and the possibility of such an adulteration was accepted as part of the risk.

Later, it was discovered that the skin itself harbored many unseen bacteria and viruses. When a needle, no matter how sterile it had been made, punctured the skin, it could inadvertently push microbes from the dermis into nervous tissue. If this happened, a local paralysis might develop at the injection site, causing someone's arm or leg to go numb. If the body's immune system wasn't fast enough to develop antibodies to the infection, it might spread towards the spinal cord where it could do real damage.

Needless to say, physicians were loathe to admit this event. The growing body of serums and antitoxins were administered chiefly to children, and the realization they may have paralyzed —even killed—one of their patients in an attempt to protect them from a future disease was not something they were keen to face. Eventually, it became common knowledge that summertime—when the poliovirus was thought to be circulating—was a dangerous time to administer vaccines. Doctors began to wait until the season had passed, hoping their discretion and improved sterilization techniques would protect their patients from harm.

The new cause of poliomyelitis had a name—provocation polio. It could have been due to a virus or bacteria, but unlike the "natural" infections paralyzing children all over the country, this route into the central nervous system was crystal clear: A needle had punctured the skin and pushed a microbe from the dermis into the nervous tissue.

* * *

As the collection of causes of poliomyelitis was growing, the frantic hunt for a cure or prevention was narrowing. The popularity of Koch's postulates had unfortunately winnowed broad scientific research down to the quest for a single, causative virus. Even so, it was clear that funding available for poliomyelitis research was not going to be enough: the sacrifice of thousands of Rhesus monkeys was extremely expensive, and the post-World War I economic depression that had overtaken the country had hit many philanthropists hard.

Although the scope of the search would continue to shrink, the intensity and number of participants was about to explode. A new *cause célèbre* was just around the corner. He was cherished the world over, and his towering presence as the president of the United States would bring infantile paralysis front and center. What the 123 residents of Rutland, Vermont and the 6,000 dead of 1916 could not accomplish, this man would.

Chapter Twenty-Nine

Campobello, 1921

IT WAS THE SUMMER OF 1921, AND just off the coast of Maine, Franklin Delano Roosevelt and several others were traveling aboard the 141 foot *Sabalo*, steaming towards his summer home on the island of Campobello. He could have taken the train from New York, but it was not like him. The rail would provide a monotonous journey that would give his restless mind hours to brood. Roosevelt, a former senator of New York, had not only just lost his bid for the vice presidency of the United States but was being dragged into a scandal associated with his tenure as Assistant Secretary of the Navy. The uncertainty of a three-day journey at sea might at least keep him occupied until he was able to see his family already gathered on the island.

As they neared the end of their trek, foul weather struck hard, laying down a thick layer of fog which gave the ship's captain pause. Having spent much of his life sailing throughout the bays and inlets of the island, Roosevelt calmly took the helm and safely piloted the large yacht into Welshpool Harbor, less than a mile from his home.

A tender came out to meet them, loading both passenger and their trunks of luggage for the short trip to the Roosevelt's dock. Later that afternoon, Roosevelt—ever eager to entertain his children—returned with some of his family in order that they could board the great vessel on which he had arrived. After a tour and some drinks, his children returned home while the adults stayed on for dinner.

It is tempting to envision a scene such as this played out in absolute luxury—well-mannered children in embroidered smocking galavanting around the shiny teak decks of a grand ship. As the first *royal* family of the United States, the Roosevelt name inevitably conveys a sense of resplendent grandeur. The reality was much different. The *Sabalo* was a Navy patrol ship hastily converted into a passenger vessel and offered few amenities. And while the Roosevelt's cottage was no hovel, it had no electricity, little plumbing, and a finicky boiler that could provide a bit of hot water—so long as storms washed enough driftwood onto the beach to keep it fired.

Franklin's wife Eleanor was unpretentious in her own way and insisted she—rather than the housekeeper—make the journey across the bay each week to the mainland town of Eastport to pick up groceries for her family. In preparation for her husband's arrival, it's likely she would have picked up a few quarts of fresh blueberries. They were plentifully available in August as just across the border, Maine's Washington County was the world's largest producer, and her famous blueberry pudding was one of Roosevelt's favorite delicacies.

* * *

The next day, Roosevelt took his guests out on the tender. While demonstrating how to fish for cod, he slipped from the boat and into the water. Though he was able to grab the side before being completely submerged, he noted something distinct—perhaps a harbinger of what was to come:

> *I'd never felt anything so cold as that water! I hardly went under, hardly wet my head, because I still had hold of the tender, but the water was so cold it seemed paralyzing. This must have been the icy shock in comparison to the heat of the August sun and the heat of the tender's engine.*[60]

The next day, Roosevelt took his children sailing around Campobello and spotted a fire on a nearby island. Ever the thrill-seeker, he made towards the smoke and they spent the next several hours extinguishing the blaze. After returning home, exhausted, Roosevelt challenged his children to a race across the island. Some two miles away was Campobello's largest lake—a strange, landlocked body of fresh-water just a hundred feet from the ocean. After donning their bathing suits, they took off towards their favorite swimming hole. Taking their father's lead, they swam across the lake, took a quick plunge in the icy waves of the Atlantic, then jogged down the dirt path back home.

Back at the cottage, Roosevelt stayed on the porch to read the newspaper—too tired to even change out of his bathing suit. As dinner was served, he realized he had no appetite and instead went straight to bed. The next morning, on Thursday, as he arose, he realized that one of his legs was "lagging" behind the other. He was able to get up and shave, but before long, it was clear his other leg was beginning to fail. Stabbing pains began to surface throughout his body, and his temperature began to rise. A nearby doctor was called in, but was unable to offer any specific diagnosis.

By Friday, Roosevelt could no longer stand up. His skin became sensitive to the slightest touch, and his clothes and bedsheets could create excruciating pain. Later that night, the paralysis had ascended so drastically he could not even grasp a pencil in his hands.

A second doctor was found—some one-hundred miles away—and brought back to the island in hopes of saving Roosevelt's life. His vital spirit began to fade as the paralysis continued to rise. Regardless, the visiting doctor diagnosed him with a blood clot in his spinal cord and suggested he get copious massage on his affected limbs—an excruciating plan of action that would have driven anyone else mad.

With his condition worsening, evidence began to suggest he might be suffering from infantile paralysis. This would have been a confusing diagnosis for a thirty-nine-year-old man, let alone a person of Roosevelt's lineage. Poliomyelitis was thought to be solely the province of children, particularly immigrant children—if one spoke about such things privately. For a stalwart individual like Roosevelt, who could sail for hours, fight fires, and run across islands for sport, the possibility of being permanently handicapped was devastating. Eventually, an expert physician from Boston was called up and made the diagnosis that everyone feared: poliomyelitis. Infantile paralysis. A real possibility that Roosevelt would never walk again.

After a few days, the paralysis had reached his face but miraculously had spared the muscles of respiration. He would live, although in what capacity no one knew. His grand political aspirations—his "conviction that in the great drama in history, with Almighty God its author and producer, he had been assigned a major role"[61]—would be shaken to its core. He had lost the vice presidency to a Republican challenger, his name was being dragged through the mud of tabloid newspapers, and his hand was currently too weak to even attempt his signature.

* * *

On September 16, 1921, the New York Times ran a front page story that shocked the country:

F. D. ROOSEVELT ILL OF POLIOMYELITIS

Despite his family's best efforts to hide the affliction, word of his suffering had gotten out, even as he lay in pain in his cottage bed. He was carried in a custom-made stretcher from his home into a boat, laid on the floor, out of the eyes of curious onlookers. It was announced his boat would arrive at a particular dock on the mainland, a purposeful diversion that would allow them to carry his flaccid frame into a waiting train car without any photos being taken.

It was inevitable the public would discover his condition. The revelation that Roosevelt had come down with poliomyelitis was a bolt from the blue, a startling wake-up call for anyone who had considered themselves immune to the disease. If he could be stricken with infantile paralysis, then perhaps anyone could. The illness—which had existed in relative obscurity alongside more prominent diseases—now had its poster child, and no one would ever think of poliomyelitis the same.

Chapter Thirty

Roosevelt

A QUESTION IS OFTEN RAISED REGARDING WHETHER Roosevelt actually contracted "polio." In light of the understanding that poliomyelitis—as originally described—can be caused by many things, it is probable that he did have numerous lesions in the gray matter of his spinal column. Very few things can cause the symptoms he experienced besides such an injury. But when a modern reader asks, they are intending to question whether Roosevelt suffered from the effects of the *poliovirus* infecting his nervous system.

Unfortunately, it is impossible to answer that question. A conclusive diagnosis of poliovirus infection within the nervous system is difficult, even with today's technology. Based on clinical symptoms alone—or even a spinal tap to examine the pressure and clarity of the spinal fluid—one could not say for sure what caused the problem.

Nevertheless, there are many facts mentioned in Roosevelt's story that do point towards something other than a poliovirus infection. The most glaring problem is the sequence in which FDR experienced his symptoms. The standard course of events is a fever, headache, and possibly some nausea. This is the effect of the body fighting off an enterovirus infection in the gut—a common illness that anyone may experience from year to year.

After a few days, the virus is able to traverse the body's numerous layers of protection and enter into the bottom of the spinal cord, where lesions produced by inflammation can create paralysis in the legs. This specific sequence has become the hallmark of a paralytic enterovirus infection—not even the poliovirus specifically, but any of them—cocksackie, echovirus, D86, etc. Roosevelt seemed to experience a much different chain of events. A fever did arrive, but only after he had already began to suffer weakness in his legs. Perhaps his vigorous lifestyle precluded him from even noticing the effects of sickness days earlier, but for someone to suffer from paralysis *then* a fever would not be common with an enterovirus infection.

His particular mention of the extraordinary cold of the water when he fell off the boat sounds suspiciously like the beginnings of *hyperesthesia*, or extreme skin sensitivity that became so troublesome for him. While pin and needle sensations can occur if the poliovirus is able to infect the nervous system, its proclivity for disrupting the back of the spinal cord—where sensory information is conducted—is rare.

Additionally, what Roosevelt experienced was far beyond the prickled skin of hyperesthesia—he underwent debilitating pain at the slightest movement or touch, a phenomenon that is decidedly unlike polio.

Additionally, it is extremely unlikely that a 39-year-old man had yet to encounter—and develop immunity to—the poliovirus. Although islands seemed to offer a protective element from infection, Roosevelt spent much of his life away from Campobello. His children did develop a fever, runny nose, and soreness in their neck—something that is very indicative of an infection of some kind, but none of them suffered the numbness, paralysis, or hyperesthesia their father did. The fact that they came down with something suggests there might have been a microbe involved.

Knowing that Roosevelt was extremely fond of fruits and berries—many of which were grown in the world-famous barrens of Washington county just miles from his home—makes the case for lead arsenate poisoning a distinct possibility. The acute pain and sensitivity he experienced is in line with such an event. The extreme physical exertion he experienced in the hours leading up to his attack is commonly associated with metal toxicity events—including poliomyelitis—and is perhaps a phenomenon which may help explain how both metals and microbes are able to migrate out of the intestinal tract and into the spinal cord.

Finally, FDR continued to experience strange symptoms. A month after the initial onset of paralysis, he developed an eye problem so acute he feared he would lose his sight—another symptom more frequently associated with arsenic or lead poisoning than polio. Neither he nor his doctors would have been aware of the danger of pesticide toxicity, and it's likely he would have continued eating lead arsenate-containing fruits.

It is clear that Roosevelt developed lesions on his spinal cord. Although doctors of that era would have no way of knowing what had caused his suffering, a modern interpretation of the events does not point towards a poliovirus —or any enterovirus—infection. Perhaps there was a microbial component involved, as evidenced by his children coming down with a mild illness, but regardless, to hazard a guess on the source of his suffering is pure conjecture. Poliomyelitis, in the classical sense of the word, yes—Roosevelt most likely had developed such lesions along his spinal cord. A diagnosis of polio, meaning an infection of the central nervous system specifically by the poliovirus? Probably not. Some have suggested Guillan-Barré syndrome, but again, a definitive diagnosis is impossible to make.

* * *

No statesman would suffer the catastrophic events of the summer of 1921 and interpret them as signs of future distinction, yet somehow, Roosevelt did—so much so that he would eventually become president for over twelve years, guiding the country out of the Great Depression and through the hardships of the second World War.

During that time, people with disabilities were not viewed with the same kindness or compassion they might receive today. Because of the hardships and economic suffering of that era, everyone was expected to contribute. Those who couldn't hold gainful employment in some capacity were often viewed as a burden to society. F.D.R. was able to fight past many naysayers —including his mother, who insisted he retire from public service and live out his days as a quiet "country gentleman"—to run for the highest office in the land and win.

While serving as president, Roosevelt's public appearances were carefully staged to avoid portraying him as a "cripple." He wore painful braces that locked his knees and ankles in place and was able to walk short distances by carefully throwing his legs in front of him. Through cooperation from a willing press, pictures of his withered legs or him in a wheel chair were few and far between—an unspoken agreement unlikely to be honored today. Regardless, his candor regarding the difficulties of his condition and perpetual advocacy for children suffering from infantile paralysis drove funding into research at a measure no other disease—or poster child—could match.

Chapter Thirty-One

Airplanes

Any bug that eats lead
Will soon need a casket;
Children should skin
The fruit in the basket.[62]

Roosevelt's poliomyelitis was wholly attributed to the work of an unseen microbe, but nevertheless, concerns about the toxicity of lead arsenate began to grow. Although isolated stories of poisoning and death occasionally appeared throughout the United States, the British imported huge quantities of American apples and were not so forgiving when their own citizens became sick. With threats of tariffs and embargo, they were able to force American growers to produce fruit with a lower amount of residue. Meanwhile, those in the United States were unknowingly eating produce with much higher levels of pesticide than what was allowed to ship outside the country.

Another problem arose. It had always been assumed that pesticides were excreted from the body quickly. The issue of chronic toxicity was very rarely discussed, but in the mid-1920s, the concept of problems resulting from the gradual accumulation of lead arsenate began to surface. A lone physiologist wrote of his concern, fearing that arsenic and lead could create "lowered resistance to disease, lessened efficiency, and shortening of life." In an early reference to the possibilities of chronic toxicity, he said, "we may not… consume enough lead and arsenic in our fruit to produce acute poisoning in tissue injury, but who is there to say that the slow assimilation of metallic poisons brought about by modern industry is without danger and ultimate injury?"[63]

They did not know it at the time, but metals such as lead or arsenic are not readily excreted from the body. The kidneys are not designed to filter out such toxins, and as a result, metals tend to accumulate in organs. Researchers begin tying arsenic toxicity to neuritis, cancer, and eczema in children—even going so far as to link the skin condition to elevated amounts of arsenic found in their mother's breastmilk. Regardless, most who grew fruit and vegetables for a living believed that the concerns over pesticide toxicity were overblown.

In 1927, the "Hunt Committee" gathered for a "Conference on the Effects of Arsenic and Lead and Food," a huge meeting intended to address the issue of pesticides and lead arsenate toxicity once and for all. Scientists, toxicologists, and other industry experts presented their most recent evidence and discussed the potential for both acute and long-term damage from these new pesticides. Growers and industry insiders were ecstatic with the result of the meeting:

> *The conferees are of the opinion that evidence of prevalence of lead and arsenic poisoning from the ingestion of fruits and vegetables sprayed with insecticide and fungicides is scanty and unconvincing.*

The amount of arsenic tolerance proposed by the committee was over twice what other countries would allow. It was clear the government's role in protecting the public was being subverted by industry insiders and the close connections they held with those they were supposed to monitor. The agricultural industry armed itself by funding aggressive lobbyists and research with results that were all but guaranteed to favor more spraying.

Unsurprisingly, scientists begin to defend the safety of lead arsenate aggressively, producing research for hire at a steady clip. T.J. Talbert, a horticulturalist from the University of Missouri, published a series of papers attempting to put both farmers and consumers at ease about the supposed toxicity of the pesticide. He said, "There is little likelihood of a human consuming as spray residue on apples sprayed and handled in the usual manner, enough arsenic either at one time or over an extended period to be injurious."[64] This suggestion—bought and paid for by industry growers—would prove woefully inadequate over the next few years.

As enthusiasm for the pesticide continued to accelerate, the end of World War I brought the surplus of a new contraption that would promote the use of lead arsenate beyond what anyone thought possible—the airplane. As hostilities ceased in Europe, the abundance of aircraft and pilots returning home from the war was put to use by the agricultural industry, surveying huge fields from far above, inspecting them for signs of insect damage.

Although the gypsy moth had extended its range far beyond New England, the state of Ohio had a different invader to deal with—the sphinx moth. Based on the success of their aerial observations, it was decided to try administering lead arsenate from above. Lieutenant John Macready piloted a trainer aircraft outfitted with a hopper of powdered lead arsenate slung onto the side. Another person rode along and could control dispersal of the pesticide by opening a small door on the side of the container.

Macready and his passenger made several passes over a large swath of Catalpa trees and the sphinx moth larvae which were feasting upon them. Follow-up reports indicated the application of lead arsenate was a huge success. According to those in attendance, Macready "accomplished in 54 seconds what would have taken two men with a wagon and a team of mules a week to do."[65]

Word of their triumph spread rapidly and before long, World War I planes were being outfitted with purpose built nozzles and tanks—converted into flying pesticide spraying machines. All over the country, farmers (and out-of-work military pilots) rejoiced over this newly discovered technique.

For almost 30 years, lead arsenate had been painstakingly applied by hand, sprinkled from garden barrel hoses, or sprayed from horse-drawn carts with pressurized tanks. More recently, it had been slathered onto livestock through the use of cattle dips.

At the conclusion of World War I, the era of cropdusting had arrived, and lead arsenate, already the most popular pesticide in the country by far, had a new method of application that would bring its effects—both positive and negative—far beyond the fruit growing states of the North.

Chapter Thirty-Two

Boston, 1928

IT WAS OCTOBER, 1928 AT THE BOSTON Children's Hospital. A girl, eight years old, was suffering the worst effects of poliomyelitis—the muscles that allowed her to breathe were failing. Like so many others, she had probably woken up one morning and noticed a distinct weakness in her legs. Her parents would have watched in horror as the immobilization slowly crept up her spine and into her arms over the next few days. Unfortunately, the paralysis had continued into her rib cage. Without the ability to breathe on her own, she would soon die.

A detailed account of just such an event was given in a 1912 study on poliomyelitis. Although heart wrenching to read, it provides a clear context as to the horror of death caused by infantile paralysis:

> *The typical clinical picture is that of one with a clear, alert, sensorium fighting for every breath until he is literally suffocated. In fatal cases there is usually a pause after the acute onset of the paralysis. There may be one or two days without any definite increase in paralysis, but it is noticeable that the children are not doing so well as those that will eventually recover. Often the respiration is more rapid and a trifle more difficult than the degree of paralysis warrants. They are frequently unusually excitable and irritable. Then the paralysis may begin to increase. A laryngeal disturbance with hoarseness, aphonia, or difficulty in swallowing may be the first evidence of the spreading lesion. If the intercostals are still active the movement of the chest becomes less marked. If the diaphragm has hitherto been intact, its movement, as represented by the abdominal wall, becomes weaker, or there is an asymmetric movement suggesting a paralysis of one side of the diaphragm. The alae nasi dilate*[i] *with inspiration, and the accessory muscles of respiration of the neck come into play. As the diaphragm weakens, the neck muscles become more and more prominent until it seems as if the whole work of breathing depended on them. The head is thrown back, and with every breath the lower jaw is pushed downward and forward in an attempt to get air. Meanwhile the lungs may have remained perfectly clear until the very end, or a few hours before death coarse moist râles*[ii] *may accumulate, an edema suggesting vasomotor paralysis. Heart sounds have been audible for as much as five minutes after breathing stopped. Several times a characteristic arrhythmia has set in for the last few hours of life. It*

i. *The base of the nostrils.*
ii. *Abnormal rattling noises heard by examining the lungs.*

is interesting that in one case, in association with the institution of artificial respiration and a lessening of cyanosis,[iii] *the irregularity of heart action completely disappeared.*

With the onset of respiratory difficulty, it seems as if the children were suddenly awakened and made to realize the struggle before them. One sees a sleepy baby become all at once wide awake, high strung, alert to the matter in hand, and this is, breathing. The whole mind and body appeared to be concentrated on respiration. The child gives the impression of one who has a fight on his hands and knows perfectly well how to manage it. Instinctively he husbands his strength, refuses food, and speaks when necessary with few words. One little child, aged 4, unable to move but with a mind that seemed to take in the whole situation, said abruptly to the nurse, between her hard taken breaths, "Turn me over." "Scratch my nostril," and then, to the doctor, "Let me alone doctor." "Don't touch my chest."

Pressure on the chest, tight neck-bands, anything that obstructs easy respiration is immediately resented. The child is nervous, fearful, and dreads being left alone. He often shows an instinctive appreciation for the specially efficient nurse. The mouth becomes filled with frothy saliva which the child is unable to swallow, so he collects it between his lips and waits for the nurse to wipe it away. The pallor is distinctive, the lips blue, cyanosis absent, and sweating profuse. The mind becomes dull, unconsciousness follows, and an hour or more later respiration ceases.[66]

It is not hard to imagine the absolute elation the parents of the eight-year-old girl in Boston must have felt when they were told her life might be spared this brutal ending. A professor and

---

iii. *A bluish discoloration of the skin resulting from poor circulation or inadequate oxygenation of the blood.*

engineer from the nearby Harvard School of Public Health had been working on a new device and thought it might extend—if not outright save—her life.

In 1894 Vermont, when poliomyelitis first struck the nation *en masse*, artificial respiration was a topic which had not been thoroughly explored. The subject was mainly discussed alongside aiding drowning victims or problematic childbirths. Midwives who delivered babies not yet breathing would first try "slapping the nates," otherwise known as spanking them across their buttocks. Their preferred method was breathing in a gulp of air, then exhaling into the baby's mouth or nose. Doctors weren't convinced this technique was safe, as it was thought most of the oxygen in the air was consumed with every breath. This belief would last until 1954, when Dr. James Elam first proved mouth to mouth breathing could provide enough oxygen to sustain life. It was later shown that humans breathe in an average of 20% oxygen with every breath and exhale 15% oxygen—a revelation which gave rise to the current acceptance of rescue breathing.

In the meantime, there were several different body manipulations taught in hopes of expanding and contracting the lungs. One might recognize *Schaefer's method*, a technique popularized in old cartoons when a drowning victim was placed on their stomach and the rescuer would straddle their legs and mash their lower back with all their weight, a gulp of water spewing forth from their mouth with every push. None of these exercises were very effective and because mouth-to-mouth resuscitation was thought not to work, a mechanized breathing apparatus was needed.

* * *

The first commercial positive respirator was 1907 Germany's Pulmotor machine—a small, portable device connected to a mask which fit directly over the patient's mouth and nose. Positive respiration had some dangers—the pressure of air going into people's lungs had to be carefully regulated, especially in patients who were deathly ill and could not respond to verbal commands. Too little volume and they would suffer from oxygen deprivation. Too much, and they would suffer from the effects of hyperventilation. Patients with positive respiration also could not talk with their masks on, further isolating them.

There was concern with the Pulmotor that air would inadvertently go into the stomach. Also, it relied on suction to pull air from the lungs, and there was additional worry the process might injure the delicate alveoli. Regardless, the Pulmotor was considered a short-term machine to resuscitate victims of trauma. Because many victims of poliomyelitis did not recover, they would need an artificial way to breathe that might go on for months, even years—something that was gentle and, rather than positive pressure, used the natural expansion of the chest to draw air in. They needed a negative air pressure machine, one that could create a vacuum around the chest cavity to expand the lungs and fill them with air.

* * *

Philip Drinker was an engineer in Boston and had been called in to consult on maintaining proper air temperature in a ward for premature infants at the Children's Hospital. While making the visit, he passed by another area that contained children—many of them infants—in the last hours of their fight with poliomyelitis. Roused by their horrific suffering, Drinker suggested that one of the patients in the ward might benefit from an artificial respiration machine he had developed and had safely tested his colleagues on.

At the time, respiratory failure was a growing concern for a host of reasons besides poliomyelitis. The invention of electricity had created a new hazard—often found directly in the home—that would cause electrocution for many. The car, and more specifically its odorless exhaust, carbon monoxide, would create a new generation of victims—completely unaware of the invisible peril and its ability to asphyxiate.

The Consolidated Gas Company of New York had become so concerned with deaths from respiratory failure that its Committee on Resuscitation and Related Activities had given Drinker substantial funding to develop a device that could safely and reliably provide respiration for those who were near death from a traumatic event.

As someone who had long studied the effects of carbon monoxide poisoning, Drinker was well aware of the difficulties with positive respiration. Drawing on inspiration from earlier designs, he set out to build an effective negative respiration machine and had the Machine Shop at the Harvard Medical School help him construct a large metal tank. On one end, a patient's head protruded through an air-tight rubber collar. Electrical pumps could alternate between creating negative and positive pressure within the tank, an effect which would expand and contract their lungs, forcing the exchange of fresh oxygen.

Drinker tried the device on several colleagues and was pleased with the amount of force the machine could generate. Those who experienced a few minutes inside the machine were taken aback at their inability to hold their breath, such was the force of the device. Controls were added to adjust the rate of breathing, as well as the temperature of air inside the tank so the patient would not get unduly hot.

There was a major problem with the initial prototype, however—it was loud. Later versions would use an electric motor which could quietly push and pull on a large diaphragm at the end of the tank, but Drinker's design used two blowers that would have sounded more like landscapers at work than artificial respiration.

* * *

When the eight-year-old girl and her parents first saw Drinker's respirator, they likely felt more fear and panic than relief. The prototype was constructed of as much wood as iron, and the blaring roar of two electric blowers had to have been disconcerting. Both doctor and parents would have realized her death was imminent without a miracle intervention and so despite their apprehensions, a rubber gasket was secured around the girl's neck, and she was locked into the tank.

With the machine switched on, she would have felt immediate relief. Besides paralysis of the muscles—some of which provided for the contraction and expansion of her lungs —there was nothing wrong with her. Without the intense physical and mental effort required for breathing, she could relax—probably for the first time in days. Drinker reported,

"During the time the child was in the respirator, she was able to talk, sleep, and take nourishment while the pumps were running."[67]

Although modern accounts of this first true test of Drinker's device often tell of how the girl miraculously recovered within minutes of being placed inside, the actual outcome was not so uplifting. The machine was able to sustain her life for 5 days, but she eventually succumbed to cardiac failure attributed to extensive bronchopneumonia—a common end for anyone who could no longer effectively cough fluid or mucus buildup from their lungs.

Despite the eight-year-old girl's tragic death, the fact that Drinker's respirator had kept her alive for 122 hours was promising. She wasn't suffering during that time. She was able to talk with her parents and slept comfortably. The pneumonia could possibly have been averted—perhaps a future treatment would prevent infections.

The iron and wood machine reverberating throughout the halls of the Boston Children's Hospital may have been unable to save its first patient, but finally, after 34 years of gruesome asphyxiations, the threat of death from poliomyelitis was lifting.

Chapter Thirty-Three

Robot Breather

"I BREATHE," BARRETT HOYT WHISPERED QUIETLY TO Philip Drinker, the engineer standing beside his invention in the lobby of the hospital.

Hoyt was twenty-two years old, a student and manager of the Harvard hockey team and was nearly dead. A few days earlier, he had noticed a weakness in his left leg and arm. Within hours, paralysis had spread to his chest as signs of troubled breathing appeared.

When the doctor finally arrived, Hoyt's neck muscles stood out "like iron bands."[68] The doctor gave Hoyt just two hours to live and in a last ditch attempt to save his life, phoned a nearby hospital and asked them to ready their Drinker respirator. With his head covered in sweat and his lips turning blue, Hoyt's condition was so precarious the doctor asked the respirator to be moved into the hospital lobby so not a second would be wasted.

Once the ambulance arrived at the hospital, Hoyt was rushed directly into the machine, with Drinker himself—called in from his laboratory nearby—waiting to take over. As soon as it was turned on, the young man's red blood cells began filling with oxygen, and relief washed over him.

"I breathe," was all he could muster. The pallor left his face, and for the first time in many days, he was able to sleep. The next morning, they removed him from the tank, and his respiration immediately faltered. With the little breath he could muster, he begged them to put him back in. For the next few days, Hoyt was wheeled in and out of the machine in an attempt to gauge if any strength had returned to his body. Eventually, after the device had kept him breathing for months, he was able to breathe unassisted and left the hospital.

It was a miracle he survived. In any other town across the country, Hoyt would have died—another victim claimed by poliomyelitis. But by sheer luck, he lived in Boston and was seen by a doctor who was familiar with Philip Drinker's device. While not everyone could recover the use of their muscles after poliomyelitis, no other artificial respiration device would have been able to safely sustain their life long enough to find out.

* * *

Word of Drinker's respirator spread quickly. With a public growing increasingly anxious over the menace of infantile paralysis—and the promise of life-saving serums so far turning up empty—physicians, journalists, and public health officials were eager to provide anxious parents any glimmer of hope they could find.

The earliest epidemics had been limited to rural areas of the country—a geographical anomaly long gone. When the outbreaks began happening in large cities, they were still limited to the northern states. But now, as the 1930s approached and cropdusting brought the application of lead arsenate far beyond the range of the gypsy, coddling and sphinx moths, it was clear that poliomyelitis could happen anywhere.

All over the country, it seemed that nothing could slow the inexorable arrival of infantile paralysis each summer. The most severe isolation and quarantine measures had little affect on its spread. The techniques for treating children who had been struck had not improved beyond massage and exercise or boards and braces.

If anything, the threat of poliomyelitis was growing and Drinker's respirator made its entrance at just the right time. Manufacture of the machines commenced, and newspapers across the country began to fill with daily updates of the few lucky souls whose lives were sustained by the rare machine.

> *NURSE KEPT ALIVE BY 'DRINKER RESPIRATOR'*
> *For Six Days and Nights Life of France McGann Has Been Prolonged*

Wealthy benefactors gave money to local hospitals, ensuring their city would not go without a machine. Los Angeles ordered one, Chicago ordered two, and controversy erupted in San Francisco when its lone machine was needed simultaneously by two dying poliomyelitis patients—a 25-year-old married father of a fourteen-month-old and an unmarried, childless 30-year-old woman. The man, an athlete, was thought to have a better chance of surviving and so received a stay in the machine by doctors, no doubt riddled with guilt. After deciding to place the father into the machine, "Miss McCulloch died a short time later, in extreme agony," a report stated, bluntly.[69]

Editors attempted to capture the imagination of the enraptured public and angled for just the right phrase to describe the miracle device. "Mechanical Lungs," "Breathing Machine," "Robot Breather," and "Lung Robot" were some of the colorful labels used in place of the more pedestrian "Drinker's Respirator." Eventually, reports of the miraculous machine dropped references to both Drinker and robots and settled on a distinctively 1930s American title, the "Iron Lung."

Within a few years, Jack Emerson, the son of New York City's Health Commissioner Haven Emerson, developed an improved version of Drinker's device. It was more comfortable for the patient, as it featured a mattress on which they could lay, and had windows and access ports along the side through which nurses could tend to patients without having to remove them. Perhaps more importantly, it was lighter, quieter and cheaper to manufacture than Drinker's, opening the door for less affluent hospitals to purchase one.

Progress would come slowly. By 1936, there were only 222 iron lungs in the entire world.[70] While the expense and complexity of the iron lung would ensure its rarity outside of large metropolitan areas for the next few decades, it offered a thread of hope that was badly needed. Even though the summer epidemics might continue, and paralysis might provide a lifetime of handicap, at least some of the gruesome deaths from the asphyxiation of infantile paralysis might be consigned to the past.

Chapter Thirty-Four

Los Angeles, 1934

By 1934, Franklin Delano Roosevelt had pushed through the stigma of his disabilities and was elected President. John Dillinger, the infamous American gangster, escaped from an Indiana jail, only to commit another bank robbery days later while Bonnie Parker and Clyde Barrow's brazen crime spree across the country came to an ignominious end under a hail of gunfire in Black Lake, Louisiana. Despite the public's obsession with these real-life criminals, they were more entranced by the miraculous accounts of poliomyelitis patients and their struggle to survive inside iron lungs.

As summer approached, the nation's public health officials dutifully checked their local papers, visited area hospitals, and made daily phone calls to doctors—all in hopes of identifying a potential outbreak of infantile paralysis in its earliest stages. Their options to contain it were pitifully few. Isolation and quarantine would be strictly enforced, but with so many asymptomatic carriers of disease on the loose, these draconian separations were more for show than anything.

A remedy that had become fashionable at the time was to pool the blood of survivors of poliomyelitis attacks and administer it to children who showed any of its early warning signs. The Los Angeles County Hospital was ready in that regard—they had over 15 gallons of *prophylactic serum* on hand, hopeful the poliomyelitis antibodies contained within would offer enough protection to spare the little ones the worst of the paralysis.

Across the country, Simon Flexner and the scientists at the Rockefeller Institute were sacrificing dozens of Rhesus monkeys every week in an attempt to unlock the mysteries of poliomyelitis. They had narrowed their focus to a single causative agent—the poliovirus, but even so, a possible vaccine for even that seemed years away. The way in which the poliovirus infection was spread? Unknown. The way in which the poliovirus reached the nervous system? Unknown. Many features of infantile paralysis were no more clearly understood then than they had been decades earlier. Regardless, two other groups who had been experimenting with a poliovirus vaccine began to make waves across the scientific world as they claimed their products were nearly complete. For the summer of 1934, the country would have to wait.

On May 18th, an article appeared in the Los Angeles Times.

HEALTH WAR ORDERED ON PARALYSIS: Dr. Parrish Authorized to Take Needed Steps to Halt Poliomyelitis Spread.[71]

George Parrish, the city's Health Officer noticed a large spike in suspected cases of infantile paralysis. By May he would have normally seen 20 cases. This year, there had been 61. For anyone who had dedicated their life to public health, such a realization would have created a rush of anxiety and fear. Most entered the field out of a sense of duty to the public good, and poliomyelitis outbreaks gave them the opportunity of a lifetime to prove their mettle. At the same time, the spotlight being shone upon health officers during poliomyelitis outbreaks—particularly in large cities—was intense. Could they control the spread? Could their hospitals cope? Could the public's faith in public institutions be maintained?

As June approached, it became clear to Parrish that they might be at the beginning of a large poliomyelitis epidemic. The recently opened Los Angeles County Hospital was buzzing with nearly 100 patients per day suspected of having developed infantile paralysis. Outside, the parking lot was filled with children, laying in wait on stretchers or the cars they arrived in.

But something was different that summer. The earliest poliomyelitis epidemics were located in mainly rural areas. In the 1900s, city centers began to experience more of the illness. While children had been a constant target of paralysis, adults seemed remarkably immune. Within that group, another class of people seemed even more protected—doctors and nurses. Whether it was their constant exposure to microbes, or their heightened sense of hygiene, one could not say, but if the outbreaks of infantile paralysis that had occurred in the previous forty years demonstrated anything, it was that medical staff were a distinct collection of people who had nothing to fear from the disease. In a curious turn of events, health care workers in Los Angeles began to be attacked.

> *HEALTH MAN STRICKEN*
>
> *Pronounced to be suffering from infantile paralysis, Hugh Bumiller, assistant chief sanitary inspector for the county health department, yesterday morning was taken to the General Hospital, where it was found necessary to place him in the Drinker respirator, according to Dr. J. L. Pomeroy, county health officer.*[72]

While it was out of the ordinary for an adult to suffer paralysis so severe they needed artificial respiration to sustain their life, it was extraordinarily odd such an adult worked in the medical field. Apparently, he was not the first. The June 16th article also mentioned Dr. Mary Bigler, "...who for many years has been head of the contagious diseases department at the hospital and who has worked night and day with poliomyelitis patients during the past three weeks, was stricken with the disease Thursday."[73] Fortunately, her condition was considered good.

A doctor—who as head of contagious diseases had surely been exposed to microbes galore—being stricken with poliomyelitis was extremely disconcerting for those watching the epidemic unfold. After a few weeks had passed, it became clear—medical professionals, particularly those who worked at the Los Angeles County Hospital, were being targeted. Nearby Juvenile Hall, a detention center where 25 to 30 children arrived every day, not a single case of poliomyelitis was reported. Other hospitals appeared to be similarly protected.

Inside the L.A. hospital, doctors and nurses were being stricken at an alarming rate. It was unlike anything they had ever seen and contained an additional element of mystery—those that were affected often displayed symptoms markedly different than typical poliomyelitis features. Severe headaches. Twitching, cramps, and muscle aches in seemingly random parts of their body. A common complaint—extreme fatigue and intermittent muscle weakness. The most frequent symptom of poliomyelitis—paralysis—was largely gone.

With limited measures at his disposal, a single Drinker respirator for the entire city, and the promise of a vaccine still months, if not years, away, Los Angeles Health Officer George Parrish phoned the Rockefeller Institute in New York and asked for help. Simon Flexner and his scientists were happy to oblige. Opportunities for research in the 1916 outbreak had largely been squandered. The epidemic—and health infrastructure—in Los Angeles could support more exhaustive efforts to catch the virus in its tracks. Perhaps the Rockefeller Institute might be the first to have a vaccine after all.

With crates of medical gear, several cages of Rhesus monkeys, and a trunk full of clothes, Dr. Leslie T. Webster of the Rockefeller Institute and Dr. John Paul of the Yale School of Medicine boarded a train and settled in for the 4-day journey to Los Angeles.

Chapter Thirty-Five

The City of Dreams

WORD OF THE IMPENDING ARRIVAL OF SCIENTISTS from the Rockefeller Institute grew quickly. Although Los Angeles and the surrounding areas had already grown to include over two million residents, their isolation from the rest of the country was no doubt more keenly felt in regards to science and medicine. The city of dreams had quickly become known for its prolific movie studios, but Boston, New York, and Philadelphia had some of the world's greatest scientific minds. Los Angeles had so far been spared the ravages of large poliomyelitis epidemics, but now that one seemed imminent, they badly wanted the medical expertise that was so prevalent on the East Coast.

As Webster and Paul's train neared Los Angeles, they were telegrammed by an anxious Parrish. Scores of newsmen had gathered at the train station and would undoubtedly attract hundreds of onlookers as the city anxiously awaited the "science men" and their marvelous monkeys. Parrish suggested they disembark in Pasadena, beyond the prying eyes of the press. Webster and Paul agreed, but were discovered hiding at the mayor's office by eagle-eyed reporters, where they were besieged and asked for statements regarding their research. Eager to get to work, the scientists refused to make any announcements, after which the photographers began pleading with them to at least produce a few monkeys for pictures.

A week later, the scientists had set up a temporary lab and secured the services of a local "animal man" to ensure the health of their stressed monkeys. They began collecting samples from both the living and the dead and injecting nasal washings or ground-up tissue into their precious few creatures. The results were profoundly disheartening. Poliovirus seemed to be almost nowhere. Only 25% of fatal poliomyelitis cases were capable of paralyzing their monkeys. And out of thousands of nasal washings gathered from the close contacts of suspected poliomyelitis patients, they were only able to paralyze nine monkeys.

Whether he was asked to help because of this anomaly, or had planned on assisting anyway, the Mayo Clinic's Dr. Edward Rosenow, proponent of the *poliomyelitic streptococcus* bacteria, arrived in Los Angeles and made clear they weren't finding the poliovirus simply "because it wasn't there."[74] Webster, the Rockefeller Institute's scientist, wrote home to his wife and confided his worst fears:

> *No one knows how much of this disease is polio—nearly all adults—nurses and doctors still coming down—much pain and weakness—very few deaths—not nearly the amount of paralysis that one expects. So I'm covering the possibility of this being a new or somewhat different virus.*[75]

At the hospital, fear gave way to hysteria. Besides the one hundred admissions every day, more of the staff—doctors, nurses or helpers—became sickened. To confound their distress, some of the sickened hospital staff had received injections of prophylactic serum—to protect them from the threat of poliomyelitis—just before coming down with illness.

With the weight of the two million residents of Los Angeles on their shoulders, Webster and Paul worked tirelessly, day and night. Considered some of the best scientific minds available, they had travelled across the country, at great expense and with tremendous fanfare, to find polio. Instead, they were faced with the prospect of not only being unable to reliably spot signs of the poliovirus, but not having any clue as to what was happening.

A dejected Webster wrote his wife again.

> *Personally, I question whether it is polio—but that is a matter of opinion, purely... There is hysteria of the populace due to a fear of getting the disease, hysteria on the part of the profession in not daring to say a disease isn't polio and refusing the absolutely useless protective serum—that has become evident once again.*[76]

Webster and Paul had already known that the prophylactic

serum being aggressively pushed throughout the city was useless but due to professional courtesy to their colleagues, kept silent. They were in a much tighter spot regarding their current research—they simply could not publicly state the epidemic was not poliomyelitis, though many features obviously pointed elsewhere. Perhaps if they could have identified the actual cause, they would have had the professional fortitude to admit the mistake and offer up the true source as penance.

By the end of the outbreak, 1,792 residents of Los Angeles County had been definitively diagnosed with poliomyelitis. Many more had come down with an illness thought to be infantile paralysis but was eventually ascribed to something else. Incredibly, 198 of the hospital's employees had been affected—5.4 percent of physicians and almost 11 percent of the nurses. Amongst the medical staff, no one died, and only 25 deaths occurred city-wide—a remarkably low rate compared to even typical epidemics of the day. Some of the cases, particular amongst the children, clearly resembled classical poliomyelitis. But many others did not, particularly the staff at the Los Angeles County Hospital.

Much speculation has been made about the source of their suffering and its possible connection to the protective serum they received. Because just over half of the staff who were sickened received the treatment—some of them *after* the onset of their illness—it's difficult to believe they were connected. Others have mused that experimental polio vaccines being developed in New York and Philadelphia may have played a part, but they would not make an appearance on the West Coast until the next year.

The symptoms experienced by the staff of the Los Angeles

County Hospital resemble chronic lead poisoning more than anything else. Parts of the building had been newly opened and construction was likely to be ongoing. Lead paint and dust are known environmental hazards but were not likely to have triggered concern, especially given the hysteria of infantile paralysis that was at the forefront of everyone's minds. Patients who stayed for short periods of time were unaffected, as were the family members of hospital staff. The only people who seemed to be troubled were those who worked in the recently developed building every day.

No matter the cause, the panic of poliomyelitis was real, and health officials, doctors, and nurses in the city of dreams were beginning to see it in places it may have not even existed. Scientists who found themselves in the middle felt the pressure for a solution growing. The rush to develop a vaccine against the mysterious poliovirus would charge ahead, a pace at which mistakes were inevitable. Los Angeles' George Parrish didn't know it—indeed not even Webster, Paul, or Rosenow knew—but that summer, one of the experimental poliovirus treatments being developed on the East Coast had been tried on more than just monkeys. In New York, three doctors—along with the inventor himself—had submitted themselves to the first ever poliovirus vaccine. They would survive. Others would not.

Chapter Thirty-Six

Thick as Thieves

As stories of infantile paralysis filled the newspapers, some of the smaller, regional hospitals began to receive their own iron lung. A few of these events were turned into pompous spectacles, staged to improve morale—and perhaps flatter the benefactors who paid for them. The enormous respirators, decorated in gallant ribbons and bows, rolled down loading ramps to the flashes of photography and the delight of gawking parents and medical staff alike. For the mysterious disease that appeared in summer and could claim the life of the hardiest boy in town, they now had a weapon with which they could fight back—the iron lung, a marvelous contrivance that could rescue seemingly anyone from the brink of death.

Research was moving painfully slow in understanding the cause of poliomyelitis, but amongst many scientists and researchers, an ominous pall had been cast over their work. Infantile paralysis—at least in its epidemic form—had come out of nowhere to the forefront over the past few decades, but it was not the only problem. New illnesses seemed to be appearing—strange diseases for which there was no historical record of their occurrence, no explanation as to their cause, and certainly no headway being made in what might be done to prevent or treat their effects.

In 1917, a strange illness they called *Australian Disease X* appeared on the remote continent. Although the symptoms were frightening—high fever, muscular rigidity, mental confusion, and coma— half of those affected were under 5 years old, and many of them died.

The Spanish flu pandemic of 1918 had killed tens of millions, but was often accompanied with an altogether separate disease called *encephalitis lethargica*, a condition which killed over a million people on its own. This strange condition, also called *sleeping sickness*—for the catatonic state in which it would often leave its patients—spread throughout the world but has never again appeared in epidemic form.

In 1924 and 1935, thousands were killed in Asia due to an obscure illness termed *Japanese encephalitis*. Other conditions appeared, such as *serous meningitis* and *St. Louis encephalitis*. The rate at which these new diseases were appearing left many concerned—so much so that Simon Flexner, head of the Rockefeller Research Institute, addressed them directly in a presentation:

The reappearance of cases of epidemic encephalitis in Europe and America in the last few months has served to emphasize the sinister character, as well as our imperfect knowledge, of the disease. Moreover, it has served to remind us of the notable fact that within a period of about twenty years, several epidemic diseases having their chief seat of injury in the central nervous organs have prevailed widely in America and in other parts of the world.[77]

Despite their differences, all of these diseases had one thing in common—they affected the central nervous system, a component of the body which until recently had appeared immune to assault. It was an unsettling coincidence —several new diseases had emerged, roughly at the same point in history, and all of them affected the nervous system. It seemed as though the human race was becoming more and more susceptible to attack, and no one could predict when they might stop.

To add to their concern, a rash of similar new diseases began to appear in animals. Mice could develop an infection from the *TO virus* and exhibit symptoms resembling the paralysis of poliomyelitis, something they called *mouse encephalomyelitis*. Pigs also began to experience paralysis from something they termed *Teschen's* disease.

The beginning of the rise in nervous disorders can be tracked through the 1800s by the ascent of "Nervine" rest homes and fainting rooms. During this time, doctors began to treat a new nervous system illness they called neurasthenia. By the end of the century, when Paris green and lead arsenate began to be sprayed aggressively, the isolated cases of neurological disorders would become widespread epidemics.

If the causes of poliomyelitis were in fact due in part to the effects of ingested pesticides or medicinal metals, it would stand to reason there might be other related issues. Because a routine enterovirus infection could migrate into the spinal cord due to a gut suffering the effects of acute lead arsenate intake, it would seem possible that other previously trivial microbes might also be given the ability to cause problems by this same mechanism.

With the spate of epidemics of the new nervous system diseases which Flexner mentioned, it was clear—the central nervous system was no longer protected—for humans *or* animals. Something significant had changed. These were not diseases that had existed elsewhere and had been able to jump continents due to increases in international travel. They were a new type of illness that appeared to have previously never existed. And more worryingly, all of them seemed perfectly capable of breaching the previously impenetrable nervous system of their hosts.

Chapter Thirty-Seven

1935

It was within this cloud of unknowing that scientists around the country had been racing forward to develop a vaccine for what they suspected was the single cause for infantile paralysis. By 1935 several attempts at creating a poliovirus vaccine had been attempted. It had long been recognized that if someone survived an infectious attack, they were likely to never suffer from its affects again. With this in mind, researchers tried to create immunity artificially by injecting ground-up spinal cord tissue of convalescing monkeys in increasing dosages. Test animals who were able to survive were assumed to have immunity and might receive an injection of the poliovirus directly into their brain—an assault which no one was likely to survive.

It is helpful to remember that at that time, and indeed for almost the next 20 years, scientists were working completely blind. Although the invention of the electron microscope was already happening, the ability to actually see the poliovirus would not happen until 1953. The only way scientists would even assume they were working with a true poliovirus was by observing the effects of injecting it into Rhesus macaque monkeys. Some injections would produce reliably fatal results, while others seemed to consistently be more innocuous. Because of this affect, it was assumed that there might be different strains of the poliovirus—some more virulent than others.

Given the technical limitations of their experiments, and considering there were several other enteroviruses that were capable of creating paralysis, it's remarkable they were able to detect early on that there were in fact multiple types of poliovirus.

Another problem would stymy vaccine development—they were still uncertain as to the route of infection. Many still believed the nasal passage was the portal of entry into the central nervous system, while others were sure the mosquito—possibly even the horsefly—was spreading the disease. Because their test animals could not reliably be infected via oral administration, they were injected with the poliovirus to test if their immunization techniques had worked. This method was certain to produce misleading results, as the gut was the natural route of infection. Someone who had developed immunity within their intestines might still succumb to a poliovirus infection if administered directly into their brain.

The earliest attempts at a poliovirus vaccine used heat in order to inactivate the microbe. Other chemicals were applied, such as aluminum hydroxide and carbolic acid. In the 1930s, a physician named Dr. Maurice Brodie, began experimenting with a potential polio vaccine that used formalin as the inactivating agent. Through many different attempts, he eventually arrived at a process through which he was confident the poliovirus could be inactivated, yet still induce immunity in those it was administered.

By the summer of 1935, Brodie was so confident in his vaccine that he and a few other doctors administered the injection to themselves. This was an undoubtedly poorly constructed safety trial, as most adults were likely to have already developed complete poliovirus immunity. Nevertheless, with their lives intact and test monkeys showing positive effects from the injections, Brodie moved into a serious trial of the vaccine involving over 3,000 children.

No one would be willing to purposefully challenge the injected children with a poliovirus infection to see if it worked, so Brodie and his colleagues tried to time the trial in an area where a polio epidemic was likely to happen. As summer approached, Brodie and his team leveraged strong relationships with local public health officials in California, Virginia, and North Carolina, to administer the vaccine through various pediatric outlets.

Initially, the results of the trial seemed promising. Brodie reported that "formalin inactivated virus is probably a perfectly safe vaccine in as much as no harmful affects have developed after more than 3,000 inoculations."[78]

Perhaps their close relationships with those who

administered the trials helped provide cover, as it was clear that 3,000 inoculations had not been safely administered. After the trials had ended, a scientist from the Rockefeller Institute mentioned there *had* been cases of poliomyelitis after receiving the Brodie vaccine. Whether any of the children had died from their injuries is unclear, but whatever the case, the Brodie vaccine was shelved and would never be tried again.

At that same time, a scientist named Dr. John A. Kolmer was feverishly working on a different approach to a potential poliovirus vaccine. Rather than trying to kill the virus with formalin, he attempted to weaken it in a series of chemical baths that to this day remains a mystery. After administering it to himself and his two children, he also moved forward to test the safety of the vaccine in a larger group of kids. Although numbers are hard to come by, Kolmer's vaccine was distributed to at least 582 physicians across 36 states. It is thought that several thousand children received his polio vaccine that summer, and this time the results were more clear. Children were developing poliomyelitis directly after the vaccine at rates as high as one in 1,000. Many of them died.

While Brodie's vaccine gave cause for alarm, Kolmer's vaccine was worse—far too dangerous to be administered to anyone. The rush to stop the threat of infantile paralysis had cost dozens of children their lives. Brodie apparently took his own life several years later, and Kolmer's poliovirus efforts would disappear into obscurity. The failures of the two 1935 poliovirus trials would put a tremendous damper on efforts to develop a vaccine and the physician's motto of *Primum non nocere*—first, do no harm—was only just beginning to be put to the test.

Chapter Thirty-Eight

Arch Enemies

ANY BUG THAT EATS LEAD
Will soon need a casket;
Children should skin
The fruit in the basket.[79]

By the late 1930s, concerns over the potential toxicity of lead arsenate had grown to a fevered pitch. A book entitled *100,000,000 Guinea Pigs* had been released and chronicled the deceptive techniques and contaminants manufacturers were using all over the country to sell their wares at higher profits. Other muckraking journalists uncovered the influence industry had over the FDA and consumers began to realize that the amounts of lead arsenate allowed on their food was definitively not as safe as they had been told. The mail room at the FDA begin to flood with complaints:

> *In the interest of the children of America in their foods. My heart goes out to them. For many years they have never had natural foods to eat. Natural foods raised under natural law, God's law... No more arsenical spray of contamination. Poison in every form should be prohibited.*

In a letter of unintended irony, a Miami woman wrote to Roosevelt's wife, the first lady:

> *Asking your kind indulgence, I want to tell you that I thank God for having placed your noble husband at the head of our government...I realize the great problems he has before him, and therefore hesitate to write to him regarding the one which I'm about to present to you, although I cannot believe that others must've brought the same subject to his attention.*
>
> *While chemists the world over are feverishly working to concoct poisonous gases for the wholesale destruction of their fellow-men—which all right minded people condemn, our farmers and horticulturalists are poisoning our own people with deadly insecticides. Compounds of arsenic are in common use, and one of these—lead arsenite[sic]—is sold in enormous quantities...It seems to me the chemists of the country should be set to work to discover an effective insecticide that would be harmless to humanity. And law should be made putting a stop to the use of these poisonous applications...And surely something should be done to stop the use of these poisons on our fruits and vegetables, from the effects of which many people have lost their lives.*[80]

While Roosevelt's condition was most likely tied directly to the harmful effects of lead arsenate, the sentiment of this woman was felt all over the nation. In an attempt to boost productivity and lower the cost of food, farmers had clearly built a bridge too far. Another book struck an even more raw nerve. *40,000,000 Guinea Pig Children* focused on the health dangers of the sprays and their effects on children—specifically, their love of fresh fruit.

As *100,000,000 Guinea Pigs* stated, it was clear to the American public:

> *...government officials have... Suppressed important information on the arsenic hazard and have resisted in every way the opening up with the question to discussion in the interest of Public Safety. The government has acknowledged the hazards of excessive consumption of arsenic residues; it has permitted residues large enough to constitute a serious health hazard; yet we cannot find it has ordered one word of warning to the public, or even so much as suggested mildly that apples and pears be peeled before they are eaten.*[81]

While Kolmer and Brodie were conducting their vaccine trials, the FDA began to relent and cracks in the veneer appeared. On a 1935 radio broadcast of "Uncle Sam at Your Service," the announcer opined:

> *A is for Arsenate—*
> *Lead, if you please,*
> *Protector of apples*
> *From arch enemies.*

But he was not done. He stated that lead arsenate could not only kill insects, but if left to remain on produce sold to consumers, it could cause chronic illness. "Fortunately for us, the growers can keep down to a safe limit the amount of the poisons occurring on their fruits and vegetables," he offered to nervous consumers as comfort.

It was an incredible admission and directly from the FDA. The program was an attempt to thread the needle—to address the concerns of a public growing increasingly aware of the problems of lead arsenate, while keeping farmers and their industry representatives happy at the same time.

Another document came out in 1936, one that might have been considered the nail in the coffin for lead arsenate as it came directly from an FDA employee. Information officer Ruth deForest Lamb had seen shocking collections of reports documenting the problems created—not only by contaminated food supplies—but also by the drug and cosmetic industries. Her book, called *American Chamber of Horrors*, clearly documented the scope of the problem, was a bestseller, and was nearly converted into a theatrical release by 20th Century Fox. Within, Lamb told story after story of children sickened or killed by eating fruit contaminated with lead arsenate.

The public became furious at having been lied to for so many years. Parents all over the country wondered what ill effects their children might be suffering from. The tempest which began brewing after the release of Ruth deForest Lamb's book would not be quelled.

By the end of the 1930s, lead arsenate, the pesticide which had its inauspicious beginning 40 years earlier—after the inadvertent release of the gypsy moth in Boston, Massachusetts

—was finally being acknowledged for its toxicity. The clouds of war had been gathering over Europe yet again, and with lead arsenate being pushed out of the picture, a new pesticide was needed. Science would again deliver, this time with something even more insidious.

Chapter Thirty-Nine

1939

THE YEAR WAS 1939. AFTER MANY YEARS of experiments, the American Medical Association finally gave its seal of approval to the practice of treating *dementia paralytica* and other syphilis related disorders with tryparsamide injections, an arsenic compound developed at the Rockefeller Institute. While debates were raging about the potential toxicity of lead arsenate in the nation's food supply, the age of metallic medicine would "not go gentle into that good night."[i]

MGM studios released "The Wizard of Oz" to the American public, rapt with wonder for its dazzling sets and

i. A reference to Dylan Thomas' 1951 poem "Do not go gentle into that good night."

Technicolor imagery. It would be nominated for six Academy awards but would lose the Best Picture category to another legendary work from that year, "Gone with the Wind." In Europe, the mood was not so jubilant. Reports began to surface that Nazi Germany had invaded Poland, and the warnings of many—so seemingly dire before—had come to light. Adolf Hitler had fomented not only the burning desire among the German people for *lebensraum*, but the materiél by which they could claim it.

Years earlier, another invasion had begun. The potato beetle —which had survived the assault of Paris green as it made its westward trek across the United States—arrived in Europe. Attempts were made to ban the import of American potatoes, but with the growth of international travel, the invasion of *Leptinotarsa decemlineata* was inevitable. It had first crossed the Atlantic in the early 1920s and had been foraging across the fields and pastures of France ever since. By the late 1930s, it had become a serious threat to the potato crops of the Swiss, and research was undertaken to find a more effective insecticide.

Paul Müller, a chemist working out of Basel, Switzerland, began experimenting with different formulations—searching for something which might slow the beetle's progress. By chance, he tried an obscure combination first synthesized in 1874—dichlorodiphenyl trichloroethane, also known as DDT. The chemical—nearly lost to obscurity—killed the potato beetle more effectively than anything he had ever witnessed. Even more impressive was its ability to adhere to that which it was applied. Weeks could pass—along with heavy rains—and the leaves on which the potato beetle fed would still kill them.

Müller quickly began testing the compound on other

insects and was thrilled with the results. Scientists in America —many of them pressed into service for the military—began to recommend applications of DDT amongst service members to help control typhus and malaria. As a result, in Naples, Italy, the yearly wintertime outbreak of typhus was stopped—a feat that had never happened before. In the Pacific, an entire island was sprayed to protect American soldiers from malaria:

> *For the first time in medical history an entire island in the Pacific is being sprayed with DDT. Twenty-two hours after the first planes landed on the island a nearly invisible mist of a DDT solution was settling over mosquito-breeding mangrove swamps. The spray, a mixture of DDT in oil, kills every insect on contact.*[82]

DDT was a miracle and was hailed in the press as a military weapon as important as the P-51 Mustang or the proximity fuse. It was a revelation of modern science, different than the toxic metals of old, like arsenic or lead. This synthetic chemical was made in laboratories by bespectacled men in white coats—not mixed in the field by uneducated laborers and sprayed wantonly. Its toxicity to humans was unknown and, in the jubilance of its effectiveness, was not questioned:

> *DDT is harmless by itself. When mixed with talc or kerosene it is deadly to insects but harmless to man, so far as the evidence goes. When it is thus sprinkled on clothing it retains its insecticidal power through eight washings. Sprayed on walls it will keep flies away for three months.*[83]

As the war pressed on, the services of DDT were called on

again and again. Its native form was a white powder and could be applied directly to clothing, administered with hand-pumped FLIT guns inside winter coats and down pant legs. For spraying, it was combined with the most readily available liquid in war—fuel—and dispersed from the air, free from the toxicity concerns of lead arsenate or Paris green.

Albert Sabin, a scientist who had been hard at work in developing a poliovirus vaccine, was called into service for the war effort and amidst his research began to notice curious patterns amongst the health of U.S. troops. In the Philippines, he reported on this phenomenon:

> *The Filipino population numbered over 61,000 in the area in which poliomyelitis was occurring at a high rate among American adults. While no clinical poliomyelitis was discovered among them, the circumstances left little doubt that the natives were the reservoir of the virulent virus which was infecting the Americans... This brings us to a consideration of the problem why the virulent strains of poliomyelitis virus produced little or no recognizable paralysis, even among the Filipino children, while the American troops in this particular area and time were becoming paralyzed at a rate which was at least 20 times higher than that obtaining for the troops in the United States or Europe.*[84]

DDT was initially in short supply and was mostly reserved for the Pacific theater, where the threat of malaria was a constant concern. Sabin thought it odd these troops were having outbreaks of poliomyelitis while the civilians amongst the islands they co-inhabited—not to mention American troops stationed elsewhere—did not. The scientist noted the same effect in other places, such as nearby China:

> *In 1946, while investigating an outbreak of poliomyelitis among American Marines in Tientsin, China, I was also informed by physicians in Tientsin, Peiping, and Shanghai that paralytic poliomyelitis was a most uncommon disease among Chinese children.*[85]

What started as a paralytic affliction in the rural countryside of America and Sweden had found its way into the urban cities—and had now somehow followed the American troops half way around the world. Was this just another remarkable coincidence of poliomyelitis?

For someone who has never known a life without air conditioning, it is difficult to convey the annoyance of never being able to escape the buzz or bite of insects. Even wintertime, when homes were sealed shut to keep in the heat, might bring with it huge numbers of lice, bedbugs, or fleas. In 1945, as the German forces finally appeared to be collapsing, entomologists and farmers, housewives and children—all of them eagerly awaited the end of World War Two, when the country's industrial complex might again be directed towards civilian use. Some were excited about being able to eat chocolate again, or getting new tires for their car. For many, they were looking forward to being able to see firsthand the incredible power of DDT.

They would not have to wait long.

Chapter Forty

1946

THE SUMMER MONTHS OF 1945 HAD PASSED when World War Two was finally declared over. Germany had capitulated in April, and the unconditional surrender of Japan—infamously signed aboard the USS Missouri—happened in September. By the next summer, the United States would regain her industrial footing, and DDT would take center stage.

The highly anticipated pesticide began being used everywhere against everything. Trucks equipped with industrial fogging devices would drive through neighborhoods and down public beaches, emitting mile-long clouds of DDT through which frolicking children would run, their parents no doubt ecstatic in the knowledge they would be protected from the harm of insects.

Advertisements began to appear in magazines, touting the content of DDT as their chief selling point: Contains 3% DDT! 5% DDT. 10% DDT! Sprays, powders, even DDT-infused wallpaper and paints from Sherwin-Williams became hot selling items—recommended especially for use in nurseries to protect vulnerable infants.

Archival footage of summer-time spraying clearly shows how safe the pesticide was assumed to be: Children in pools, being doused in DDT powder as they play. Youngsters at a picnic table, thick clouds of DDT wafting through their lunches as they eat. There was seemingly no limit to the amount of the insecticide that could be safely sprayed directly onto humans and anything they might touch, wear, or ingest. The military war was over, and the bugs of summer were gone—at least for now. The nation was elated with her post-war industrial might and the modern conveniences that scientific progress had wrought.

* * *

After the war, industrialized farming began at a pace the country had never seen before. The medicinal chemicals of old, arsenic, lead, cyanide, mercury, and sulfuric acid, were replaced with powerful weapons of war—the same chemicals the military had used to ensure victory over the Axis powers in Europe and Japan. Surplus planes and pilots were immediately put to use, and DDT began to fall from the skies everywhere across the United States. An excerpt from the *New Republic* gave readers a poignant glimpse into what was going on:

> *On May 23, 1945, the sun shone warmly on a large oak forest near the village of Mosco, Pennsylvania. Bird calls and songs rang through the woodland as the birds flew about feeding hungry young ones. But the forest was ill; its leaves were covered with millions of devouring gypsy moth caterpillars. Though birds ate vast numbers of the caterpillars and carried them to their newly hatched young, the horde was beyond their control.*
>
> *Early the next morning, an airplane droned over the forest dropping a fine spray of DDT in an oil solution at the rate of five pounds per acre. The effect was instantaneous. The destructive caterpillars, caught in the deadly rain, died by the thousands. On May 25, the sun rose on a forest of great silence—the silence of total death. Not a bird call broke the ominous quiet.*[86]

Interestingly, the incredible killing power of DDT was eagerly anticipated not only by farmers, but poliomyelitis researchers. More than a few scientists held onto the idea that the poliovirus was spread chiefly through the excreted stool of persons infected—asymptomatic or otherwise—and assumed that the poliovirus would eventually be shown to be spread by flies.

Research continued to indicate various flying insects were in fact capable of picking up the poliovirus from infected stool samples. Whether they were able to transmit the virus on to human hosts remained unproven. With this mode of transmission in mind, some of the earliest trials of DDT amongst civilian populations were made not in the hope of protecting crops from insects, but in the hope of protecting children from polio. It would be a grave mistake.

A trial in Hidalgo, Texas, employed heavy applications of

DDT to kill off the fly population. The DDT worked as advertised and successfully reduced their population to nearly nothing. It did not, however, do anything for the human population, where a large poliomyelitis outbreak occurred during the height of the spraying.

In fact, all across the country, children began to be struck down with paralysis at rates that had never happened before, not even during the height of lead arsenate spraying. Besides the mysterious outbreak of 1916 in New York City, the epidemics of poliomyelitis had ebbed and flowed in cities and countrysides throughout the nation—sometimes more, sometimes less. After World War Two had commenced, it became obvious that something changed as paralysis rates began to skyrocket. In 1945, there had been over 13,000 cases of polio across the U.S. By the end of summer in 1946, that number would almost double.[87]

Articles in every newspaper sounded the alarm: POLIO RISE IN TWIN CITIES. POLIO CASES IN THE U.S. UP 71% THIS YEAR. OUTBREAK OF POLIO WORST SINCE 1916. The American public, still recovering from the hardships of the Second World War, watched in horror as the mysterious illness appeared again to take the lives of their children—an unseen enemy that attacked Americans on her own soil in a terrifying way the Germans and Japanese had never been able to.

In areas which appeared to be spared from the epidemic, hospitals rushed their iron lungs to places of need. With the nagging suspicion that insects could be spreading the disease, planes were called in—the "Flying Flit Guns of the Skies"—over towns experiencing outbreaks to annihilate any potential spread from insects with showers of DDT. Nothing seemed capable of slowing the spread of paralysis and unfortunately, besides the artificial respiration provided by the mechanical breathers, medicine had little else to offer besides massage, hydrotherapy, and braces.

The National Foundation for Infantile Paralysis, a charity which Roosevelt himself had helped launch, was running out of money. Through the generous donations of citizens, the group had seen to it that no family suffering the effects of poliomyelitis would worry about hospital care. By the fall of 1946, it had drained its coffers of nearly $4 million dollars and predicted it might need $24 million for the next year.

It had been more than forty years since the presence of the poliovirus was first detected, but the promise of a cure or preventative vaccine seemed as distant as it ever had. Simon Flexner, the Rockefeller Institute's charismatic director who was considered by most to be the world's leading expert on infantile paralysis, died at the age of 83. He had spent a lifetime fighting germs—chief amongst them the poliovirus—but would not be able to see the efforts of his work come to fruition.

In Campobello, a granite cairn was erected in memory of Franklin Delano Roosevelt, the poliomyelitis victim who had fought through debilitating paralysis to become a four-term president of the United States during one of the most tumultuous periods in history. The illness had nearly claimed his life at 39 years old, but the man who had become the face of infantile paralysis the world over would survive another twenty-four years, finally succumbing to a stroke just one month before the German surrender in May of 1945.

Two of the greatest figures in the history of poliomyelitis had passed away without a glimmer of hope for a cure and at a time when cases of the illness were skyrocketing. The specter of Brodie and Kolmer's experimental poliovirus vaccines still hung like a cloud over anyone who suggested another trial might be in order. While scientists were still befuddled by the transmission route of the infection, they were united in its cause—nearly all of them agreed that the poliovirus was causing the paralysis that had become so prevalent since the end of the war.

But not everyone was convinced. In 1947, a physician in New York began noticing a new illness that he and his colleagues had never seen before. Like Charles Caverly had done in 1894 Vermont, he began to document the particulars of the phenomenon and submitted a paper to his peers in an attempt to understand what was happening. The report was published in the American Journal of Digestive Diseases and mentioned symptoms which sounded remarkably similar to poliomyelitis. Within the article, he made an uncomfortable suggestion as to the source of the problem: dichlorodiphenyl trichloroethane, or DDT.

Chapter Forty-One

Virus X

In December of 1947, most in Los Angeles had forgotten about the baffling outbreak of 1935 when reports began to surface of a strange, new disease:

> *A mysterious "virus x" has stricken one of every 10 persons in Los Angeles during the last six weeks reports City Health Officer Dr. George M. Uhl.*
>
> *He said more than 200,000 cases have been reported, but there have been no fatalities.*
>
> *It has hit adults and children equally, with attacks lasting from three to seven days. Victims suffer from chills and fever, cramps, nausea and pains. It's similar in some symptoms to influenza.*
>
> *Apparently highly communicable, the virus has yet to be put to*

> *laboratory test but Dr. Uhl expressed the opinion it was not the same as Q fever, another mysterious malady being investigated by state health authorities.*[88]

At the astonishing rate of one out of every ten, no one seemed immune from the illness. Bing Crosby, Eroll Flynn, and Micky Rooney were all stricken with the puzzling constellation of symptoms doctors had never seen before. Even starlet Marilyn Monroe announced she had come down with "Virus X" during a risqué photoshoot, proclaiming, "I now keep my clothes on and I feel better."[89]

As months passed, it became clear the suffering was not confined to Los Angeles. People in Austin, Texas, began to encounter the illness, as did those in Arizona and Pennsylvania. Just as the country began to experience some of the worst infantile paralysis epidemics on record, a new disease had surfaced and was sickening both children and adults everywhere.

Although certain aspects of the illness resembled the flu, many did not:

> *Acute gastroenteritis occurs with nausea, vomiting, abdominal pain and diarrhea... Coryza,*[i] *cough and persistent sore throat are often common, followed by a persistent or recurrent feeling of a "lump" in the throat; Pain in the joints, generalized muscle weakness and exhausting fatigue are usual; the latter are often so severe in the acute stage as to be described by some patients as "paralysis..." areas of skin become exquisitely hyper-sensitive and after a few days this hyperesthesia disappears only to recur*

---

i. *Runny nose.*

elsewhere, or irregular numbness, tingling sensations... Erratic fibrillary twitching of voluntary muscles is common. Usually there is diminution of vibratory sense in the extremities.[90]

If the hyper-sensitive skin and exhausting fatigue did not remind them of many of the early case descriptions of infantile paralysis, the muscle weakness—so acute it was described as "paralysis"—should certainly have struck a familiar note. No matter its resemblance to influenza, it was obvious the illness involved dysfunction within the central nervous system.

Deaths associated with Virus X were reported, and in one of many eery parallels to the 1894 Vermont outbreak, animals also began to come down with the illness. The American public, already anxious with the recent increase in poliomyelitis, demanded answers.

Health officials went on the offensive. Some of them claimed that Virus X was nothing new, and in fact had always existed in one form or another under different names. Other scientists claimed the illness was nothing more than a form of the influenza virus and even began offering what they called vaccines to the public for Virus X. More wary individuals might have realized the vaccine was actually just a protective serum, collected from the blood of individuals who had ostensibly survived an infection, but regardless, it was clear that a new disease had emerged.

A physician in New York named Morton Biskind had first noticed the symptoms among his own patients in 1947 and began investigating the potential cause of the illness. It didn't take him long to conclude the nature of the disease might not be microbial at all.

> *The high incidence, the usual absence of a febrile reaction, the persistence and erratic recurrence of the symptoms, the lack of observable inflammatory lesions, and the resistance even to palliative therapy, suggested an intoxication rather than an infection.*[91]

Biskind stated the obvious suspect—DDT. Virus X had surfaced in the U.S. just months after the war had ended—when the pesticide was first used. The toxicological effects of DDT were nearly identical to Virus X: a runny nose, abdominal pain, joint pain, and extreme muscle weakness. The list of equivalent symptoms ran a page long, and Biskind suggested it was foolish to suppose that a chemical—known to be toxic, even in minute amounts to insects and animals—would not be so in man.

Articles appeared in papers throughout the world claiming "Virus X caused by DDT Poisoning." A Pulitzer Prize-winning author named Louis Bromfield jumped on board and began promulgating the theory that DDT—and possibly lead arsenate—might have been contributed to Virus X *and* infantile paralysis. Bromfield's appearances and Biskind's article in the *American Journal of Digestive Diseases* landed like bombshells.

The public was terrified at the spate of nervous diseases recently so prevalent, but was even more crestfallen by the thought that their cherished pesticide might be doing real harm. DDT, the miracle of science—which had freed them from the curse of so many insects—had been taken into their homes and administered directly onto—and into—their children. The pesticide had become an invaluable tool for raising infants safely—as faithfully depended on then as many might regard childhood vaccines today.

The realization that cattle were being treated aggressively with DDT in such a way it was showing up in infant milk created real panic. Government agencies and health officials rushed in to assuage nervous parent's fears, making broad statements as to DDT's inherent safety—if used properly—in both man and animal. The U.S. Public Health Service, along with the FDA, tried to calm them:

> *Statements that DDT is responsible for causing the so-called 'virus X disease' in man and X-disease of cattle are totally without foundation... Both of these diseases were recognized before the use of DDT as an insecticide.*[92]

Whether they were purposefully misleading the public or not about the sudden appearance of Virus X is unknown, but from reading accounts of the day, one gets a sense that the age old claims of "it's the dose that makes the poison" were beginning to wear thin. Children, and now even adults, were getting sick. DDT was raining down from above and below. It was dispensed automatically inside restaurants and scattered inside lunch boxes. It was sprinkled on mattresses and inside baseball caps. The doses did not matter anymore. DDT was everywhere.

Chapter Forty-Two

1952

THE YEARS AFTER THE WAR CONTINUED TO get worse. 1951 had been particularly tough for poliomyelitis—over 28,000 people had been stricken, with 1,551 of them dead. As the summer of 1952 approached, the National Infantile Paralysis Foundation, in coordination with the New York Public School superintendent, printed 1,400,000 leaflets to be distributed around the city in hopes of preventing another outbreak. Among the precautionary measures:

Let children continue to play with their usual companions.

Have them wash their hands before eating.

See that they use their own eating utensils and toilet articles and that they are always clean.

> *Pay special attention to a headache, fever, sore throat, upset stomach, sore muscles and stiffness of the neck and back.*
>
> *Call a doctor at once should any member of the family develop such symptoms, put the patient to bed and keep others away from him.*[93]

A particular admonishment stood out as health officials were no doubt aware of the dangers of provocation polio and tonsillectomies:

> *Seek a doctor's advice about nose and throat operations, inoculations and teeth extractions during the polio season.*[94]

In many states, unusually heavy spring rains created thousands of extra breeding grounds for mosquitoes. In Chicago, millions of crickets descended upon the city in nearly biblical proportions. All over the country, cities and towns reacted with more spraying as fogging trucks poured into neighborhood streets, leaving clouds of DDT in their wake.

An additional concern was affecting the way in which the pesticide was being applied. In the few short years that DDT had been available to U.S. citizens, some of the insects it was being used against had developed resistance to its nefarious effects. The housefly, in particular, seemed completely immune from harm.

Rather than experimenting with a different chemical, many entomologists advised increasing the concentration of the pesticide, far above and beyond what many would have considered safe. For the control of chinch bugs, one newspaper article recommended that 11 pounds of DDT be used per 1,000 square feet. This meant that on a half acre residential property, almost 240 pounds of DDT powder would need to be applied to have the desired effect—twice, if necessary.[95] A USDA report indicated that a single application of DDT could continue to kill insects up to five years later—a statement possibly seen as *braggadocio* by some and a shameful admission by others.

By July, it was apparent things were appallingly bad. The numbers of people being diagnosed with poliomyelitis were higher than any the country had ever experienced. In Syracuse, Thomas B. Turner Jr., chairman of the polio fund drive, would succumb to bulbar polio, following his brother-in-law just a year earlier. In Queens, a 20-year-old woman in critical condition with poliomyelitis symptoms and a kidney infection was removed from an iron lung in order to deliver a five-pound, four-ounce baby. In Rahway, New Jersey, where just weeks earlier massive DDT efforts had been rolled out to control the exploding mosquito population, Mrs. Ida La Fauci, 27, and her son Thomas, 6, were transferred to the local children's home with bulbar polio. He would survive—she would not.

Individual accounts of death were horrible, but a troubling new phenomenon emerged. In the past, the epidemiology of poliomyelitis had confused many because it often affected only the strongest child within a family, sparing many weaker siblings. In the 1916 New York City outbreak, only 5 percent of families experienced more than one case. In 1952, entire families were stricken down.

In Taylor, Wisconsin, Mrs. Hjornevik and her husband watched in horror as five of their eight children were stricken. Their oldest, Beatrice, 20 years old, would die. In San Antonio,

Texas, an article mentioned a similar circumstance:

> *Little Josephine Perl had to play alone today. Her six brothers and sisters are in the polio ward of a San Antonio hospital. So are two of the 13-year-old girls' playmates—one of them a cousin.*
>
> *The six children of Mr. and Mrs. Paul Perl, a farm couple from the Stonewall Community about 75 miles west of Austin.*
>
> *Dayton Perl, 14, was admitted Aug. 26. Last Tuesday four more entered—Daniel, 15; Paul Jr., 11; George, 10, and Elaine Frances, 9. The sixth, Dorothy, 6 was isolated Thursday.*
>
> *Late last night the hospital report on all of them was "unchanged."*[96]

In Iowa, Joe and Clara Thiel were taking no chances with their large family and ordered their children to stay away from the local swimming hole. They even purchased special polio insurance and made sure to mention to reporters they had sprayed extra DDT to keep away flies. By the time the summer was over, eleven of their fourteen children had come down with poliomyelitis. All would survive, with only two of them apparently suffering any lingering paralysis.

Outside of Milwaukee, a family of six would not be so lucky. Their oldest child, a 17-year-old high school football player was rushed to the hospital after complaining of "severe headache and pain and weakness of his right arm and shoulder." He was placed on antibiotics and intravenous fluids but would die later that night. His four-year-old sister complained of a headache and stiff neck the following day. She, too, was rushed to the hospital and given the same treatment. Despite little discomfort or trouble with breathing, she was dead by nightfall. The next three days, two more siblings would suffer the same fate—headaches, stiff necks, a hospital visit with antibiotics and intravenous fluids, then death. It was a tragic story of poliomyelitis that few could comprehend—particularly disturbing because of the speed at which they were killed. All of them had experienced mild symptoms but were gone within hours.

Stories like this played out again and again, particularly in the farm belt states of Iowa, Kansas, and Minnesota. Iron lungs were flown around the country to areas of need—North Carolina sent three towards Iowa on a military transport plane and Bedford, Massachusetts, sent their four respirators westward in case they were necessary. In the last week of August, over 3,500 new cases were reported—the single biggest 7-day total in the nation's history. Past experience suggested the numbers would go down in the following weeks but instead, they went up—and continued to rise for the next five weeks, each one breaking the record of the previous. It wasn't until October that the number of new cases finally crested and the true scope of what had happened was evident.

* * *

Besides entire families being stricken, another disturbing pattern emerged—more people were suffering the effects of bulbar poliomyelitis, the rarest and often most deadly form. For many that summer, gone was the typical "ascending paralysis" others had experienced in the past—weakness in the legs that slowly moved up through the abdomen and arms. In 1952, many were experiencing acute cranial nerve dysfunction—

trouble with speaking, swallowing, or sudden respiratory failure. Although this type of poliomyelitis had been associated with tonsillectomies, it seemed to have become more prevalent.

The way in which DDT was applied may have had something to do with it. Previously, lead arsenate was the pesticide of choice and was sprayed onto much of what people ate. As a result, it was ingested and did most of its damage in the intestines—an area located adjacent to the portion of the spinal cord which controlled the legs. DDT was administered much more liberally. Not only was it sprayed from above by airplanes, it was dusted directly onto humans, much like any bug repellant might be used today, where it could be absorbed by the skin.

Profuse applications of DDT were common during the summer months, and as such, may have provided multiple pathways into the nervous system—ingested, absorbed, even inhaled. Insects, with decidedly different anatomy than humans, could be quickly dispatched just by getting DDT on their feet. Birds were dying by the hundreds of thousands from eating caterpillars which had consumed DDT-covered leaves. It is unsurprising that humans—purposefully consuming the pesticide in these ways—would suffer. The irony these very applications were often being used in a desperate attempt to stave off poliomyelitis in children is unfortunately lost on most.

Another procedure—this one performed by doctors themselves—might explain some of the increase, particularly the bulbar variety. Penicillin was first discovered in 1928. Its true potential languished until the 1940s, when techniques for its manufacture improved to the point large-scale applications were possible. As an antibiotic, its ability to stop bacterial infections was astounding and was immediately put to use—both in the United States and the war efforts abroad.

Although infantile paralysis was thought to be caused by a virus, penicillin—which could only work miracles in certain bacterial infections—became one of the go-to treatments for anyone suspected of coming down with the illness. Physicians had few options available to them for medical care, and with parents anxious for them to do something—anything—to help their children, painful injections of the antibiotic might be administered daily, even every few hours, in hopes of lessening the effects of the illness. Unfortunately, if the child was truly suffering the effects of a viral infection, the shots would not have helped in the slightest.

Some forms of the antibiotic injections contained strange ingredients. Penicillin was thought to be metabolized too quickly in the body, and as a result, ingredients such as peanut oil and aluminum were added to extend the duration of its effects. These components—the peanut oil in particular—made the solution extremely viscous and difficult to administer without a large gauge needle.

The fortitude required by doctors to administer these agonizing injections—not to mention that of the nurses required to immobilize the terrified children several times a day—should not be underestimated. Regardless, in children suffering the effects of a viral infection or DDT poisoning—possibly both—the additional injection of metals such as aluminum under extreme duress.[i] might explain why the

---

i. A much more thorough exploration of this hypothesis is covered in *Crooked:Man-made Disease Explained.*

cranial nerves seemed so often targeted in the post-World War Two epidemics.

Additionally, the shadow of Rosenow's *poliomyelitic streptococcus* bacteria continues to haunt this particularly deadly chapter of poliomyelitis. The seemingly miraculous ability for penicillin to kill bacteria was also capable of creating intracellular bacteria as well—strange mutant forms which could infect the body in ways the immune system was incapable of controlling. As so many were treated with frequent penicillin injections during this time, it is difficult not to believe they may have had some tangential association.

* * *

In November, as the last cases of infantile paralysis were finally tailing off, parents whose children were spared breathed another sigh of relief. The final count was tallied and published for all to see—57,879 people had been diagnosed with polio and 3,145 of them had died, a shocking amount that had more than doubled the previous year's total.[97] The scattershot pattern in which poliomyelitis struck caused additional concern. Gone were the isolated cases of the 1800s. Gone were the disparate epidemics of the early 1900s. Polio was everywhere, striking both young and old, individuals and families, with seemingly no rhyme or reason, and certainly no end in sight.

Chapter Forty-Three

Fade Out

In the United States, 1952 ushered in another few changes. The number of insects developing resistance to DDT had accelerated as many began to notice the pesticide no longer worked as it had in the past—no matter the amount employed. It had become a useless deterrent on house flies and even mosquitoes seemed to be immune to its effects. More troubling were the rumored associations between Virus X and DDT. Already on alert from reports of cattle poisoning and contamination of infant milk, the general public's perception of the chemical began to decline—clearly visible in bug repellant advertisements in *Life* magazine which began to feature such selling points as "DDT-Free!" and "Contains no DDT!"

Although agricultural applications of DDT would continue a few years longer, the habit of dusting the pesticide directly onto one's children—or their lunch—fell out of favor. Ever since the end of the Second World War, its toxic effects had been suspected—and tolerated—because of its remarkable ability to kill. With its lethality in doubt, nervous mothers quickly began looking for a potentially safer and more effective substitute. At the same time, rather than frolicking in the clouds of DDT wafting down their streets, children learned to avoid the fogging trucks and hid inside until the air had cleared.

The dire warnings of Arthur Kallet's *100,000,000 Guinea Pigs* and Rachel Palmer's *40,000,000 Guinea Pig Children*—ignored for so long by government agencies and growers alike—were finally beginning to resonate with consumers. Lead arsenate was increasingly avoided by growers, and the arsenic and mercuric medicines so heavily favored by physicians had nearly disappeared. Even Steedman's Teething Powder, the mercuric medicine trusted for over 140 years—to purge the bowels of teething infants—announced it would begin using a new formula, this time without the mercury. Perhaps the era of what had first surfaced over one hundred years earlier as *teething paralysis* was finally drawing to a close.

* * *

As the gypsy moth continued its spread beyond New England, the great Adirondack mountains—with few oaks the insect preferred—served as a natural barrier. Combined with its own efforts, the Agriculture Department described its achievement in controlling the moth's expansion as "outstanding restriction of distribution and damage."[98] Fears that the gypsy moth would make it to the Appalachians and decimate the tree population there were cast aside—for a short while.

Although consumers were rapidly abandoning the pesticide, the siren song of DDT held too much promise for commercial growers to resist. The housefly and mosquito may have developed immunity to its effects, but other pests were still affected by it. And so the Agriculture Department announced a new program—not to control or restrict the gypsy moth, but to eradicate it completely. Millions of acres would be sprayed, indiscriminately from planes above. Although the range of the gypsy moth was limited to heavily forested ares, nowhere would be off limits—including densely populated towns like Long Island, where it was claimed they faced the imminent "threat of infestation from the New York City metropolitan area."[99]

DDT, mixed with diesel fuel, was dropped from the skies over Pennsylvania, New Jersey, Michigan and New York. Ponds, marshes, even suburban neighborhoods were sprayed with impunity, killing both insects and animals wherever it fell. Long Island residents sought an injunction to stop the spraying—a case which went all the way to the Supreme Court, where its review was refused. In Westchester County, New York, Mrs. Wilhelmine Waller begged officials not to spray her 200-acre dairy farm, even offering to have her entire property checked for gypsy moths. Despite promises her land would not be sprayed, it received two coatings from above in addition to the drift from nearby pastures. Within 48 hours, her cow's milk was tested and found to contain 14 parts per million of DDT. She notified the county Health Department, who seemed unconcerned and said nothing about withholding it from public consumption.

Scenes such as this continued to play out across the huge swaths of land that were sprayed. Farmers began to notice badly burned crops. Beekeepers saw their hives decimated. Bird populations plummeted to nearly zero. Other pests such as the coddling moth and fire ant were similarly targeted, and all over the United States, the devastating effects of DDT and other pesticides were clearly visible.

Scientific studies pointing towards the cumulative effects of DDT toxicity began to accumulate. Additional insects appeared to demonstrate resistance to its effects and eventually, the pesticide finally began to lose its luster—even amongst commercial farmers. The three and a half million acres which had been sprayed in the Northeast the previous year dropped to under a half of a million acres in 1958. The following years would see it drop to under 100,000 acres. And despite aggressive spraying, gypsy moths began to appear on Long Island—a harsh reminder to all those involved of the infinite complexities involved in controlling mother nature.

When Rachel Carson's *Silent Spring*—an epic exposé of the devastation pesticides were causing—hit the shelves in 1962, the public was already growing aware of the true cost of wanton spraying. England and Australia had banned or heavily restricted the use of arsenical solutions. The public had already soured on residential DDT use, and Carson's book offered any remaining doubters a stark view into its destructive nature and inspired the organization of conservation movements across the country. The use of DDT was banned in 1972, and although lead arsenate was not legally prohibited as an insecticide in the

U.S. until 1988, its use had long been abandoned.

Infantile paralysis would not strike the United States again as it had in 1952. With the prohibition of pesticides such as DDT and lead arsenate, the eventual disappearance of poliomyelitis outbreaks each summer was inevitable. The number of cases would plummet over the next few years down to nearly nothing. By the end of 1957, only 221 people died from poliomyelitis—a precipitous drop from the 3,145 just five years earlier. Swimming pools and movie theaters would remain open throughout summers, and the daily polio tallies vanished from newspapers. Mentions of Virus X, the mysterious illness that had emerged alongside the introduction of DDT, also began to evaporate. As if by magic, lead arsenate, DDT, Virus X, and poliomyelitis all began to recede into history at the exact same moment in time. Sporadic cases would continue to appear, but the epidemics which had defined infantile paralysis ever since Charles Caverly first noted the phenomenon in 1894 would never return.

Chapter Forty-Four

Chicago, 1960

It was May 1960, in Chicago. A group of scientists and physicians had gathered at the Illinois State Medical Society to discuss a troubling issue. Amongst several notable scholars and epidemiologists, was Herald R. Cox, President Elect of the Society of American Bacteriologists and a worldwide expert—and creator—of the matter at hand: poliovirus vaccines.

Many of the attendees had helped conduct trials and authored papers over the previous few years on the efficacy of the Salk vaccine—the injection many Americans had gotten in hopes of protection from poliomyelitis. Although foisted upon an adoring public, Jonas Salk was not so admired by many of his peers. The technique he used for developing a vaccine was thought to be both antiquated and dangerous. Salk would bathe poliovirus in formalin just long enough to kill—ideally without affecting its ability to create an immune response. The process had been tried unsuccessfully in 1935 and even in 1960, almost twenty five years later, the process used to ensure the poliovirus was completely inactivated still needed improvement—an unsettling fact not shared with the public.

Some of the early batches of Salk's poliovirus vaccine—destined for use in 1955—had been improperly prepared and had to be recalled. A number of laboratories had been employed for its manufacture, and the instructions relayed to them by Salk seemed to be changing by the week. Amongst the confusing production process—along with safety measures which had been relaxed—some batches were shipped containing live poliovirus. As the initial injections were being administered in various parts of the country, it became apparent the vaccine was inadvertently causing paralysis and death, the same problem which occurred in previous trials but had been carefully concealed from reporters. The public—ecstatic with the promise the shot would protect their children from harm—was deeply shaken. It would be years before Salk's injected vaccine was trusted again.

The purpose of the gathering was summarized by the reading of a quote from a Dr. Alexander Langmuir, not in attendance:

> *In a symposium on polio in New Jersey last month he stated that a current resurgence of the disease, particularly the paralytic form, provides "cause for immediate concern" and that the upward polio trend in the United States during the past two years "has been*

a sobering experience for overenthusiastic health officers and epidemiologists alike."[100]

Cases of poliomyelitis had been falling reliably each summer since 1952 but in the previous two years, starting in 1958, a distinct upward trend had been detected. The conference's moderator, Dr. Herbert Ratner, laid bare a possible cause:

> *In the fall of 1955 Dr. Langmuir had predicted that by 1957 there would be less than 100 cases of paralytic polio in the United States. As you know, four years and 300 million doses of Salk vaccine later, we had in 1959 approximately 6,000 cases of paralytic polio, 1,000 of which were in persons who had received three, four, and more shots of the Salk vaccine. So you see, expectancy of the Salk vaccine has not lived up to actuality, and Dr. Langmuir was right when he said the figures of 1959 were sobering.*[101]

A thousand people who had received at least three shots of the Salk vaccine had come down with poliomyelitis—some of them having received at least five injections. Whether they had become paralyzed from live poliovirus in the vaccine itself or from another enterovirus was not discussed, but regardless, the uptick in paralytic polio after the vaccine was being widely used was very concerning.

Another problem had become apparent: Being an enterovirus, the poliovirus replicates in the gut. Because it was injected, the Salk vaccine could only create antibodies within the bloodstream. While they believed this effect protective enough to prevent the invader from reaching the nervous system, they realized it could do nothing to prevent the intestines from harboring—and excreting—the virus by the millions.

Assuming it were true, that meant the Salk vaccine had no effect on the spread of the disease—only in the potential for it to protect from paralysis. This was a crushing realization for those intent on stamping out the poliovirus once and for all. If the Salk vaccine could only offer personal protection from paralysis, the virus would continue to proliferate and infect for eternity, requiring an equally protracted campaign of constant vaccination—something physicians were loathe to engage in.

Much was discussed at the conference about the waning efficacy of the Salk vaccine. Early trials revealed that antibodies generated by the killed poliovirus didn't last more than a few years, a shortcoming which might have explained the rise in paralytic cases. To add to their doubt, the debacle of the 1955 vaccine roll-out had prompted manufacturers to create additional protective measures—another filtration step and the incorporation of a mercury-based preservative called merthiolate—also known as thimerosal. Their influence on the efficacy of the vaccine was unknown and unlikely to be conclusively determined.

Dr. Greenberg, a biostatistician and former chairman of the Committee on Evaluation and Standards of the American Public Health Association, provided a prophetic word on the hysteria surrounding the vaccine:

> *One of the most obvious pieces of misinformation being delivered to the American public is that the 50 per cent rise in paralytic poliomyelitis in 1958 and the real accelerated increase in*

1959 have been caused by persons failing to be vaccinated. This represents a certain amount of "double talk" and an unwillingness to face facts and to evaluate the true effectiveness of the Salk vaccine. It is double talk from the standpoint of logical reasoning: If the Salk vaccine is to take credit for the decline from 1955-1957, how can those individuals who were vaccinated several years ago contribute to the increase in 1958 and 1959? Are not these persons still vaccinated?

The number of persons over two years of age in 1960 who have not been vaccinated cannot be more, and must be considerably less than the number who had no vaccination in 1957. Yet, a recent Associated Press release to warn about the impending threat referred to the idea that the "main reason is that millions of children and adults have never been vaccinated."[102]

As the conference proceeded, it was clear that many in attendance were eagerly awaiting the introduction of a completely different type of shot—a *live* poliovirus vaccine. While Salk's vaccine used chemicals to kill the virus, others were creating live, *attenuated* versions by passaging it hundreds of times through animal tissue. In this weakened state, the poliovirus could be safely administered to children orally in order to produce a true poliovirus infection—and immunity—in their gut. Several groups had already begun testing their offerings—notably Harold Cox and Albert Sabin—and felt confident the more natural method of administration would induce protection superior to that of Salk's.

The live poliovirus vaccine had its own pitfalls. Occasionally, the attenuated virus administered to children would begin to replicate and revert back to its naturally virulent state. For children with intestines wrecked by pesticides and metallic medicines, it could cause the exact same paralysis as a naturally-occurring infection. Although this was thankfully a rare occurrence, frequent administrations of the live vaccine assured the poliovirus could never be eradicated—a fact Jonas Salk was all too happy to mention.

Despite its shortcoming, a live vaccine *could* prevent an intestinal infection from the poliovirus. While the blood borne antibodies of Salk's killed vaccine were likely incapable of preventing poliomyelitis, the live poliovirus vaccine most likely could, though it would still offer protection from only one of nearly a dozen potential sources of paralysis.

In hindsight, it is unlikely any of the paralytic viruses reach the nervous system through the bloodstream. With provocation polio, the paralysis started at the site of the injection. The bulbar poliomyelitis often associated with tonsillectomies implied a similarly condensed path. In the same way, the proclivity for poliovirus infections to strike the bottom of the spinal cord adjacent to the intestines—the precise area of the body where they are harbored—suggests a direct route.

* * *

The live poliovirus vaccine of Albert Sabin won the national recommendation over that of Harold Cox, but would not be fully implemented until 1963.[i] By then, poliomyelitis had nearly disappeared from the U.S. landscape, due in large part to the dwindling presence of lead arsenate and DDT.

---

i. The initial vaccine, which protected against a single type of poliovirus, was put into use in 1961.

It wasn't just the pesticides, however. Another quirk of science and epidemiology ensured that cases of polio would plunge. Anytime an illness is studied as thoroughly as poliomyelitis was in the 1940s and 1950s, an increase in knowledge should be expected. As specifics around the nature of the disease increase, so too will the specificity of its definition. This narrowing of criteria will inevitably cause the diagnosis of fewer cases, a phenomenon Dr. Greenberg explained clearly to the gape-jawed conference:

> *If the vaccine was not as effective, one might wonder why the tremendous reduction occurred in the 1955, 1956, and 1957 reported rates. Here again, much of this reduction was a statistical artifact.*
>
> *Prior to 1954 any physician who reported paralytic poliomyelitis was doing his patient a service by way of subsidizing the cost of hospitalization and was being community-minded in reporting a communicable disease. The criterion of diagnosis at that time in most health departments followed the World Health Organization definition: "Spinal paralytic poliomyelitis: Signs and symptoms of non-paralytic poliomyelitis with the addition of partial or complete paralysis of one or more muscle groups, detected on two examinations at least 24 hours apart."*
>
> *Note that "two examinations 24 hours apart" was all that was required. Laboratory confirmation and presence of residual paralysis was not required. In 1954 the criteria were changed to conform more closely to the definition used in the 1954 field trials: residual paralysis was determined 10 to 20 days after onset of illness and again 50 to 70 days after onset. The influence of the field trials is still evident in most health departments; unless there is residual involvement at least 60 days after onset, a case of poliomyelitis is not considered paralytic.*

> *This change in definition meant that in 1955 we started reporting a new disease, namely, paralytic poliomyelitis with a longer lasting paralysis. Furthermore, diagnostic procedures have continued to be refined. Coxsackie virus infections and asceptic meningitis have been distinguished from paralytic poliomyelitis. Prior to 1954 large numbers of these cases undoubtedly were mislabeled as paralytic poliomyelitis. Thus, simply by changes in diagnostic criteria, the number of paralytic cases was predetermined to decrease in 1955-1957, whether or not any vaccine was used.*[103]

Before the introduction of the vaccine, if someone was stricken with poliomyelitis, they had to exhibit the symptoms for 24 hours to count on the register as a true case of paralytic polio. After the vaccine, it required 60 days of paralysis. With the flick of a pen, cases of paralytic polio began to instantly disappear from the record books.

It's impossible to talk about this diagnostic change without creating overtones of a conspiracy to hide the inefficacy of the Salk vaccine. This was decidedly not the case. No one was purposefully trying to manipulate the number of paralytic polio cases to make the vaccine appear to work—they were simply standardizing the diagnostic criteria to align with previous trials of the vaccine so that accurate comparisons were possible. The timing of the change—coupled with the vaccine's recall—makes it appear as though a calculated attempt was made to mislead the public. While the public *was* deliberately misled in other aspects of the vaccine's safety and efficacy, this was not a part of it.

Despite popular opinion, the much ballyhooed vaccines of

Jonas Salk or Albert Sabin likely had very little to do with the decline of polio in the United States. Although Salk's vaccine was made ready for use in 1955, the recall and resulting panic meant it would not see widespread use until a couple of years later, when poliomyelitis deaths had already plummeted from 1952's high of 3,145 to 221. Its efficacy was widely doubted by the scientific community and may not even have been capable of preventing poliomyelitis at all.

Although Sabin's vaccine did impact poliovirus infections specifically, its arrival in 1963 was too late to have had a meaningful impact when, despite its exploding population, the United States produced only 441 cases of poliomyelitis, 90 of which resulted in death.

Whether the vaccines worked or not could be considered irrelevant. Even if they worked perfectly, they were still only capable of preventing poliovirus infections and none of the other myriad causes of poliomyelitis. It is tempting to suppose that the majority of cases of paralysis in the U.S. were caused by the poliovirus specifically, but in an outbreak near Detroit, Michigan, in 1958—where over 869 people were diagnosed with polio—exhaustive studies, including fecal analysis, concluded that only 292 actually had the poliovirus.[104] Given the innocuous nature of poliovirus infections, one could not even definitively say why those 292 were sick.

* * *

Much has been made over the role of various poliovirus vaccines in the disappearance of polio, but a more careful examination of the story suggests that—at least in the United

States—their contribution was minimal. The era of metallic medicine is drawing to a close, and thankfully, most countries have moved beyond the diabolical pesticides of old. Other countries who have not still suffer mightily from infantile paralysis. India is currently the world's largest producer of DDT. While nearly 200 hundred other countries have banned its production, DDT is so ubiquitous in parts of the India it is routinely found in breast milk—an unpleasant ingredient in any infant's first meal.

Pictures of mechanized foggers, crawling down the street with children running through clouds of DDT may be thought of as relics of a bygone era in the United States, but in some countries, this hazardous practice continues to this day. It should come as no surprise that India, despite perpetual polio vaccines, struggles with various forms of infantile paralysis. This problem is so common, a newer label, *Nonpolio Acute Flaccid Paralysis (nonpolio AFP)*, was created to describe those stricken with paralysis *not* attributable to a poliovirus infection. Nonpolio AFP incidence rate has skyrocketed in the last few years, possibly due to local health officials who—under extreme pressure to get their polio numbers down by international aid organizations—are purposefully hiding polio infections within the nonpolio column.

Whatever the specific cause, it is clear that when children's intestinal health is severely compromised, paralysis will follow. Polio rates may have gone down in India, but poliomyelitis certainly has not. The crippling paralysis caused by various assaults of the central nervous system will continue to be a problem as long as the gut health of the country's children is decimated by constant pesticide exposure.

While the polio vaccine program in India may be viewed as a success by some, it has simply narrowed down one potential source of paralysis. There are still many others, and the continual spraying of pesticides have made many of the mosquitoes and other insects resistant to the effects of DDT. While it initially seemed a miracle, its long term effects on poliomyelitis and the ecology of India—indeed the world—are unknown. Perhaps unknowable.

Chapter Forty-Five

Epilogue

Amongst collections of the world's most famous photographs, the broad spectrum of human experience is clearly visible: Tragedy and suffering. Joy and elation. Wartime. Famine. Separation. Reunion. Although these compilations are not always the same, there is frequent overlap. One notable absence, missing in nearly every collection, is a picture taken in the auditorium of the Rancho Los Amigos Hospital in Los Angeles, California. It was featured in a 1953 *Life* Magazine article and would come to symbolize much about the era of America and its battle with polio.

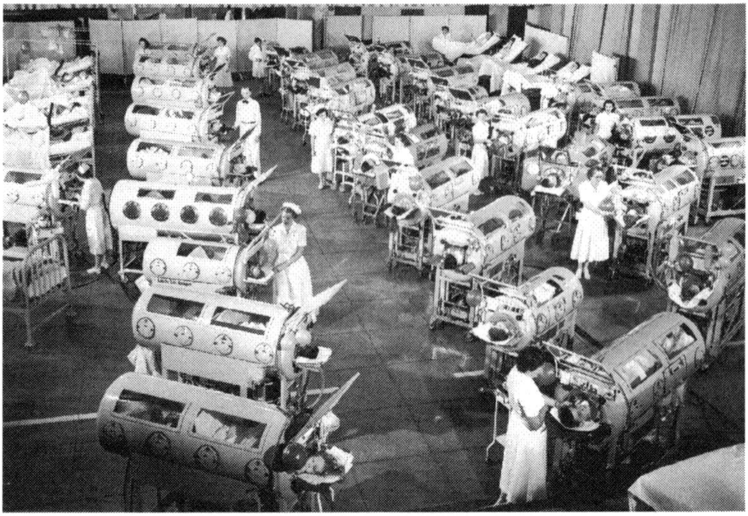

The Auditorium at Rancho Los Amigos Hospital, Los Angeles. (1953)

From atop a ladder placed on the stage, a photographer pointed their camera towards the rear of the large room, where entire rows of seating had been removed. Fifteen nurses and orderlies in starched white uniforms are spread throughout, many of them facing the camera while dutifully tending their charges. Some of the sick are convalescing in beds. The majority, however, are lying within thirty three iron lungs lined up in procession—each one adorned with several colorful balloons, their faces sometimes visible in the mirrors above.

The photograph's imagery is often invoked as dramatic testimony to both the destructive power of Mother Nature and the ingenuity of man to overcome her. The picture is powerful because it has entered into the subconscious of so many and is frequently cited as a warning to those who dare suggest vaccinations might not be as necessary as once believed. It may only be because debates on the safety and necessity of vaccinations are currently raging, but regardless, new references to the photograph and the powerful message it conveys can be read on any given day throughout the internet: Stop vaccinations and hospital wards across the country will again be filled wall to wall with dying children and their iron lungs.

No other image in any of the collections of most powerful photographs comes close to capturing the zeitgeist of a modern debate as the thirty-three iron lungs in the Rancho Los Amigos hospital does. The fact that nearly anyone can look at this picture and wax nostalgic about the miracle of vaccines—rather than the danger of ingested metals and pesticides—is an epic failure of human narcissism.

In reality, the scene depicted in *Life* magazine was a publicity stunt—a medical parade of starch and steel meant to impress upon the viewer how well equipped the United States was for dealing with future polio outbreaks. Many of the iron lungs had been recently purchased by other hospitals. Before being delivered to their final destination, they were mustered together for this once-in-a-lifetime display of medical might. A few devices—and patients—appear genuine, sporting either "Los Ranchos Amigos" lettering along their side or personal photos of loved ones above their heads. Many of the other machines appear brand new, unadorned with any accoutrement and stuffed with undoubtedly spooked volunteers.

At their peak, it has been estimated there were around 1,100 iron lungs in service in the United States. Ranchos Los Amigos featured one of the largest poliomyelitis wards in the country but is unlikely to have ever had more than a dozen of the machines in service at any given time. A similar publicity still from the Boston Hospital, home to one of the device's inventors, indicates they had seven or eight. Epidemics were few and, geographically speaking, were very far between. As such, most hospitals were lucky to have more than one. Iron lungs were expensive, not portable, and the sporadic nature of poliomyelitis outbreaks meant they would likely be sitting in storage for much of their life.

In the back left of the picture, barely visible, lie four patients whose respiration is being assisted by a cuirass—a hard plastic shell which encased their chest and could accomplish what the iron lung was capable of without the drama of entombment. This more sophisticated method of artificial respiration would never supplant the iron lung. Both of them would soon be replaced by positive pressure machines—devices that could be transported easily, operated silently, and whose only inconvenience was a small mask that covered the patient's face.

* * *

Provocation polio—an infection of the nervous system caused by an injection—does still occur. As long as nurses are thorough in their cleaning of the injection site—and manufacturers resolute in keeping their products free of contaminants or improperly treated viruses—it should not happen. But occasionally, cases of provocation polio do crop up, often visible during the late months of summer when millions of kids are receiving their shots for school—recognizable in the news with headlines like "Mystery disease paralyzes Washington child," or "Polio-like illness claims 6-

year-old." Local physicians will often have no idea as to what happened to the child, but a quick peek into the details of the case will often reveal some form of injection had been recently administered.

Although provocation polio cases are rare, the cranial nerve damage associated with bulbar poliomyelitis is much more common, visible as crooked smiles, misaligned eyes, the tilted head of torticollis or even tongue paralysis and its resulting speech disorders. Because the modern physician thinks of polio as paralysis caused specifically by the poliovirus, they are unlikely to associate these symptoms with anything nefarious. For doctors who practiced before the advent of poliovirus vaccines, they would have diagnosed children presenting these symptoms with bulbar poliomyelitis—an unsettling thought given the ubiquity of cranial nerve damage present amongst today's children.

In deference to the success of the polio vaccine, many will remark at how one never sees iron lungs today. The reality is, of course, a bit more complex. Infantile paralysis—the affliction that targeted children's legs, arms, sometimes breathing, and so common in the United States between 1894 and 1954—*is* largely gone, mostly due to the disappearance of pesticides and medicinal metals being administered to children.

But it does still occur—often hidden within other diagnoses such as acute flaccid paralysis or transverse myelitis. If paralysis threatens to disrupt someone's breathing, doctors and nurses will rush to their aid—not with the *robot breathers* of old, but with the sophisticated positive pressure machines of today. They are decidedly more effective but lack the macabre aesthetic and moniker of the iron lung. As a result, images of disembodied children of that time period, silently awaiting their fate within the mechanical breathing machines, will continue to invoke a more emotional response than the suffering of today.

* * *

The tale of polio that is told—to both children and medical students alike—does little to advance our understanding of not only what happened, but what might happen again. The account of heroic man persevering over a heartless Mother Nature needs to be corrected. Despite all the lab coats and microscopes, the March of Dimes and the Nobel prizes, the enemies were actually our own clever designs the whole time.

The widespread problems because of poliomyelitis began in 1894, Vermont, and began its decline in 1952 across the farms and swimming holes of America, as the planes and trucks began to pay closer attention to the munitions they dropped on children throughout the nation. As long as the battle of humans, their lead arsenate, and their DDT against the gypsy and codling moths remains forgotten, the parade of iron lungs at Rancho Los Amigos in 1953 will continue to haunt the dreams of mothers and fathers everywhere.

Chapter Forty-Six

Commentary

A BIT MORE DETAIL IS IN ORDER regarding the modern interpretation of the rise of poliomyelitis being due to better sanitation. This hypothesis supposes that improvements in sewage treatment procedures prevented children from safely picking up the infection while they still enjoyed the protective antibodies of their mother's breastmilk. This is a difficult hypothesis to entertain, simply for the fact the disease was called *infantile* paralysis for the majority of its history. Even well into the 1940s and 1950s, poliomyelitis—or its nickname, polio—was used interchangeably with infantile paralysis.

Even if improvements in sanitation prevented children from acquiring the infection as infants, they would have eventually acquired it later on, ostensibly at a *more* dangerous point in their life—without antibodies from breastmilk to protect them. This would suggest that paralysis should be more frequent amongst anyone *except* infants. Older children, teens and adults—having never been exposed to the poliovirus as babies—should have been the ones stricken down during the poliomyelitis epidemics, but instead, it was predominantly infants.

Additionally, rural countrysides—the hallmark locale of early epidemics—had not changed their sanitation practices in any meaningful way. In fact, many farms would continue to use an outhouse—as they had done for a hundred years—until the mid 1900s. During the earliest Vermont outbreaks, Charles Caverly spent considerable time investigating sanitation and hygiene and found few common threads between those who were struck and those who had been spared.

With the later epidemics after World War Two, when entire families—as many as eleven siblings—came down with the illness at the same time, it is difficult to believe that so many children—with fifteen years between them—had lived with sanitation good enough to avoid infection for their entire lives while at the same time lived with sanitation so poor they were all ingesting water contaminated with the excreted enterovirus of someone sick. Something else had changed after World War Two that triggered the explosion of poliomyelitis across America, and it wasn't better toilets.

Finally, this hypothesis would suggest that areas of the world now suffering the effects of polio would feature remarkable sanitation, when the opposite is true: Parts of India, Pakistan, Afghanistan, and Nigeria—where the disease still presents a tremendous challenge—are better known for their filth and contamination than well-managed latrines and efficient sewage treatment facilities.

If one believes that isolated cases of *teething paralysis* and *morning paralysis* of the 1800s—along with the epidemic outbreaks of *infantile paralysis* during the 1900s—were all due solely to reduced early-exposure to the poliovirus, despite animals and infants being the most common victims, a unified hypothesis to explain this will be difficult to come by. Despite its absurdity, the improved sanitation theory still holds the imagination of many—eager to find, most likely, a cause which doesn't implicate humans so thoroughly.

* * *

Many modern historians will claim that the effects of DDT poisoning are markedly different than polio, and they would not have been mistaken for each other. This is partially true—DDT poisoning lacks the initial fever and recovery that so often preceded paralysis of the lower extremities. It often causes tingling and pains in the joints—another symptom not commonly associated with a poliovirus infection. But just like arsenic, DDT can most definitely cause the tell-tale symptoms of poliomyelitis, as studies were indicating:

> *Degeneration and sometimes destruction of a few anterior horn cells in the thoracic and lumbar regions of the spinal cord have been noted...*[105].

Additionally, it is necessary to remember the lens through

which this type of sickness was then viewed. Besides checking the clarity and pressure of cerebrospinal fluid—a nearly useless diagnostic test—they had nothing definitive by which they could make a determination besides clinical observations. The modern poliovirus-specific description by which we think of polio is much more narrow than they would have diagnosed back then.

If someone, particularly a child, felt sick during the summer and showed any signs of dysfunction within their central nervous system—paralysis or not—they were going to be diagnosed with a poliovirus infection in the 1950s. The panic and paranoia that had taken over precluded most physicians and parents from accepting any other outcome, particularly in areas that were not used to seeing it. And as Dr. Greenberg had said at the Chicago conference, this diagnosis would guarantee free care for children courtesy of the National Infantile Paralysis Foundation.

As we now know, they most likely did have *poliomyelitis*, but whether it was caused by the infection from the poliovirus specifically was anyone's guess. As mentioned earlier, even in 1959, physicians were getting the diagnosis right only 33% of the time. This was not due to ignorance on their part, but a lack of technology combined with suspicion that each disease had a single causative factor.

In casual discussions of the disease, people will often mention a grandmother or distant relative who had polio. A conversation may come up with someone who, with the distinct limp of a withered leg, may claim they had polio. The truth is—they probably don't actually know what harmed them. They were *told* they had polio, but a definitive answer was nearly impossible for most to have received back then. They most likely had poliomyelitis—inflammation of the grey matter of the spinal cord. Whether a vaccine would have saved them from harm would be complete speculation.

* * *

An obvious question arises: Was Etienne Trouvelot and his escaped gypsy moths responsible for the emergence of poliomyelitis? The question should focus on epidemic poliomyelitis, as isolated cases of infantile paralysis, teething paralysis, and debility of the lower limbs had been occurring for decades.

Paris green had existed long before potato beetles began their eastward trek across the United States. Its transformation from ubiquitous color dye into widespread pesticide was likely inevitable. Lead arsenate, however, was the direct result of the gypsy moth invasion in Massachusetts. It is tempting to suppose the gust of wind in Trouvelot's kitchen window—had it blown inward, instead of outward—may have kept the gypsy moth egg masses under his control and the subsequent development of lead arsenate out of the diet of children around the world. Perhaps without this fortuitous sequence of events, the large epidemics of poliomyelitis—and the iron lungs that eventually accompanied them—would have never occurred.

In reality, not only would epidemic poliomyelitis have begun to occur anyway, it could have been much worse. Other invasive species were arriving frequently—some of them more harmful than the gypsy moth. Lead arsenate began to be used *en masse*, not because it was perfect, but because it worked significantly better than the existing option—Paris green. Other formulations would have continued to be tried, and in fact, the deadly insecticidal properties of DDT—first synthesized in 1874—may have been discovered in the 1892 quest to stop the gypsy moth, almost fifty years earlier. Where that path would have lead us is difficult to imagine.

The gypsy moth, the codling moth, and all of the other invasive species which had been fought so doggedly by generations of farmers continue to thrive—their legacy not only visible in the disturbed ecosystems they leave in their wake, but the withered limbs and wheelchairs which still dot the country. The pesticides created in hopes of their demise—Paris green, lead arsenate, DDT, and many others—can also be found in museums, rusty cans of poison, their skull and crossbone warnings no longer ignored.

One hundred years later, the toxic assault of lead arsenate remains, as the parents of children living in neighborhoods built on top of old apple orchards can attest. The promise of DDT continues to enchant public health officials, who occasionally suggest its prohibition be lifted to battle the imagined threats of Ebola or Zika. Like war-sick military veterans, they yearn for the good 'ole days of Flying Flit guns and fogging trucks, billowing plumes of pesticides over pastures and throughout neighborhoods. They would do well to understand the danger goes far beyond runny noses and disrupted bird populations.

The last testament to the era of poliomyelitis—the iron lung —still remains, albeit in a much different form. The mechanical breathers and steel coffins of old have been replaced with unobtrusive masks, their operation nearly silent. Although they could opt for respiration outside the machine, the last few victims of poliomyelitis have chosen to remain in their iron lungs for the rest of their lives—an understandable decision given the relationship which no doubt has formed between man and the machine that has kept them alive for decades.

* * *

The impact of Koch's postulates on the poliomyelitis story cannot be overstated. Although most modern scientists of today do not realize it, poliomyelitis was known to have several distinct causes. Laboratory experiments confirmed it. Even if one were to explain the history of the word "polio" and how poliomyelitis represented the diagnosis of a lesion within the grey matter of the spinal cord, they would be unlikely to accept the broad context in which polio used to inhabit.

The search for a single causative agent planted a seed deep within the psyche of scientists and physicians everywhere—the idea that paralytic poliomyelitis was caused by a single virus, despite all evidence to the contrary. Unfortunately, modern science has not escaped this same tunnel-vision. Where researchers of old had Koch's postulates hanging over their head, guiding their search for a lone microbe, many modern scientists are driven by a blinding quest within the genetic universe in their search for a lone strand of DNA.

Whether it is purposeful or not, both quests seem equally capable of providing scientists with an unspoken luxury—an innocuous filter which exonerates them from having to explore any potential environmental causes. The discovery of a microbe or genetic mutation makes for much more rewarding work. The implication of a disease or disorder being man-made is unlikely to generate funding or notoriety—a scientific shortcoming likely to negatively affect the lives of millions in the future.

* * *

A final thought for those reluctant to accept this portrayal of the polio story: Many will resist believing this account because of the overarching belief that history gets things right. Perhaps a few outlandish conspiracy theories are floated around here and there, but, in general, the truth will rise to the top over several years, whereupon alternate depictions—proposed so convincingly by charlatans and contrarians—will fade into obscurity.

For those that believe this to be true, the notion that the paralysis from polio was actually caused by man more so than the microbe will be difficult to embrace. They will probably feel that if this were actually the case, it would have been accepted by now.

A quick look at the Zika story which unfolded in the last several years may convince them otherwise, for the parallels to the polio story are many. In the fall of 2015, troubling reports began to surface in the northeastern sections of Brazil. Doctors were seeing an increase in the number of babies born with undersized heads, a phenomenon called microcephaly. As the months passed, it became clear that something had happened — there was a massive spike in the number of microcephaly cases. Health officials frantically searched for answers as to why this was happening. Despite locals pointing to the recent release of genetically modified mosquitoes or the aggressive pesticide spraying they had been recently subjected to, authorities were sure they had found the cause. It was a relatively unknown illness that had recently been introduced into the country – a microbe transmitted by mosquito bite called the Zika virus.

Panic overtook much of the world. People avoided traveling to South America, pregnant women aborted their babies, and a massive funding effort was undertaken in the race to develop a vaccine. Cities were sprayed from above with pesticides in an attempt to stop the *Aedes aegypti* mosquito which carried the virus, decimating bee populations in the process. Zika was spreading, and the crippling birth defects would follow along with it.

By 2016, it was clear something strange was happening. The Zika infections continued, but the birth defects did not—they nearly disappeared. The Zika virus had spread—as was predicted—but the microcephaly was absent, even from the original area from which it emerged. Initially, the frenzied research to develop a vaccine continued, but, eventually, many of the laboratories dropped their programs. It was evident that a vaccine was not going to be needed. The fear which had surrounded the initial microcephaly outbreaks—justifiably so—subsided. Mentions of Zika disappeared from the news, and besides occasional updates from global health agencies, no one is interested in the virus any longer. It is a relic of the past, a virus which went from complete obscurity—into worldwide awareness—then back to obscurity within the course of a couple of years.

Although the timeline is condensed, the Zika story closely mirrors what happened with polio: A formerly innocuous virus begins to be associated with tremendous harm, seemingly out of nowhere. The possibility of environmental causes as a contributing factor are largely ignored by health officials. A race to develop a vaccine is begun. Actions are undertaken by health officials in an attempt to stop its spread—actions which inadvertently could have made the problem worse.

There is a distinct difference between the two. With poliomyelitis, vaccines were licensed and began to be administered. The vaccines—despite their admitted inefficacy and late arrival to the scene—were declared a complete success. Parades were held and names ensconced in the great pantheon of scientific achievement.

Zika had no such program. If it did, there is little doubt that the fall in microcephaly rates would be attributed to the success of the vaccine. Claims to the contrary would be brushed aside, as would suggestions the Zika vaccine might not be necessary at all and, in fact, had little to do with the disappearance of birth defects. A search for the true cause of the spike in microcephaly that year in Brazil would be scoffed at as the wild hunt of a conspiracy theorist.

As it happened, the Zika story played out a bit differently than poliomyelitis. The environmental factor which caused the spike in 2015 was removed, and the birth defects faded away—before a vaccine arrived on the scene. If the Salk vaccine had been developed a few years later, the story of polio may have taken this exact same path. The paralysis and death that stalked children each summer in America would be largely forgotten about. But rather than attributing its disappearance to a vaccine, most would have just accepted polio—much as they have Zika—as a fluke of nature and moved on with their lives. The suggestion that their kids receive polio vaccines to protect them from paralysis would feel just as ludicrous as the suggestion that kids should receive Zika vaccines today.

Humans prefer a heroic story rather than one of dismal failure. As a result, the Zika story will never be retold. There will be no parades, no buildings named after its researchers, and books that dig deep in search of the truth will receive no awards. If there had been a heroic ending—fabricated or otherwise—we might expect a box office adaptation of the race for a vaccine. Instead, the ill-fated decision of Brazilian health officials in 2014 will be consigned to oblivion.[i]

The audacious tale of how the polio vaccine saved us from harm is so ingrained into cultural lore, it feels wrong to dispute it—indeed, many are attacked for daring to question a single detail. Because of this, the story has lived on—unsullied by those who would seek to find the truth, no matter the courage or cowardice it reveals. Perhaps the unvarnished account of polio will one day come to light and will rightly take its place in history as a portent of the arrogance of man—a change which would be most welcome. Humans will continue to prefer the heroic journey, and there are far more deserving stories to tell.

---

i. A more detailed exploration of this story can be found in *Crooked:Man-made Disease Explained.*

Selected Bibliography

ALLEN, ARTHUR. *VACCINES: THE CONTROVERSIAL STORY OF Medicine's Greatest Lifesaver*. 2007.

Allen, Will. *The War on Bugs*. (2007).

Apple, Rima D. *Mothers and Medicine: A Social History of Infant Feeding, 1890-1950*. 1987.

Atkinson, M.D., D.T. *Adenoids and Kindred Perils of School Life*. 1914.

Barry, John M. *The Great Influenza: The Epic Story of the Deadliest Plague in History*. 2005.

Beard, A.M., M.D., George M. *A Practical Treatise on Nervous Exhaustion (Neurasthenia)*. 1880.

Bookman, Debbie and Schumacher, Jim. *The Virus and the Vaccine: Contaminated Vaccine, Deadly Cancers, and Government Neglect*. 2005.

Britton, M.D., W.E. Agricultural Experiment Station, Bulletin 157. Lead Arsenate and Paris Green. 1907.

Brodie, M.D., F.A.P.H.A. and Park, M.D., F.A.P.H.A., William. *Active Immunization Against Poliomyelitis*. 1935.

Carson, Rachel. *Silent Spring*. 1962.

Caverly, M.D., Charles S. *Infantile Paralysis in Vermont*. 1924.

Chittenden, F.H. United States of Department of Agriculture, Bureau of Entomology, The Colorado Potato Beetle. 1907.

Davis, Kenneth S. FDR: The *Beckoning of Destiny, 1882– 1928; A History*. 1971.

Edwards, M.D., William A. *Cyclopædia of the Diseases of Children*. 1899.

Emerson, M.D., Haven. *The Epidemic of Poliomyelitis (Infantile Paralysis) in New York City in 1916*. 1917.

Flexner, M.D., Simon. *The Nature, Manner of Conveyance and Means of Prevention of Infantile Paralysis*. 1916.

———. The Journal of Experimental Medicine, vol. XXVIII. 1918.

———. The Nature, Manner of Conveyance and Means of Prevention of Infantile Paralysis. 1916.

Frauenthal, M.D., Henry W. and Manning, M.D., Jaclyn Van Vliet. *A Manual of Infantile Paralysis with Modern Methods of Treatment*. 1914.

Forbush, Edward H. and Fernald, A.M., Ph.D., Charles H. *The Gypsy Moth: A Report of the Work of Destroying the Insect in the Commonwealth of Massachusetts, Together with An Account of Its History and Habits Both In Massachusetts and Europe*. 1896.

Gallagher, Hugh Gregory. *FDR's Splendid Deception*. 1985.

Gilliam, A.G. *Epidemiological Study of an Epidemic, Diagnosed as*

Poliomyelitis, Occurring Among the Personnel of the Los Angeles County General Hospital During the Summer of 1934. 1937.

Greenberg, M.D., M.S.P.H., F.A.P.H.A., et. al. *The Relation Between Recent Injections and Paralytic Poliomyelitis in Children.* 1952.

Haywood, J.K., and McDonnell, C.C. U.S. Department of Agriculture, Bureau of Chemistry—Bulletin No. 131. Lead Arsenate. 1910.

Heine, Jacob Von. Beobachtungen über Lähmung Zustände der unteren Extremitäten und deren Behandlung. 1840.

———. Spinale Kinderlähmung. 1860.

Humphries, Suzanne and Bistrianyk, Roman. *Dissolving Illusions: Diseases, Vaccines, and the Forgotten History.* 2013.

Kallet, Arthur and Schlink, F. J. *100,000,000 Guinea Pigs: Dangers in Everyday Foods, Drugs and Cosmetics.* 1933.

Kessel, John. F., et. al. *Use of Serum and the Routine and Experimental Laboratory Findings in the 1934 Epidemic.* 1934.

Kolata, Gina. *Flu: The Story of the Great Influenza Pandemic of 1918 and the Search for the Virus That Caused It.* 1999.

Lavinder, C.H., *Poliomyelitis (Infantile Paralysis): The Status of the Disease in New York City and Surrounding Territory.* 1916.

———, Freeman, A.W. and Frost, W.H. *Epidemiological Studies of Poliomyelitis in New York City and the Northeastern United States During the Year 1916.* 1918.

Lehr, Teresa. *The Great Tonsil Massacre.* 2014.

Loomis, M.D., Alfred Lee and Thompson, M.D., William Gilman. *A System of Practical Medicine.* 1898.

Lovett, R. W. *The Treatment of Infantile Paralysis.* 1916.

Lovett, R. W., and Emerson, M.D., Herbert C. *The Occurrence of*

Infantile Paralysis in Massachusetts in 1908. 1909.

Maready, Forrest. *Crooked: Man-made Disease Explained: The Incredible Story of Metals, Microbes, and Medicine, Hidden Within Our Faces.* 2018

MacPhail, M.D., M.R.C.S., Andrew. *An Epidemic of "Paralysis in Children" One Hundred and Twenty Cases.* 1894.

Meier, Paul. *The Biggest Public Health Experiment Ever: The 1954 Field Trial of the Salk Poliomyelitis Vaccine.* 1957.

Millard, D.O., Frederick P. *Poliomyelitis (Infantile Paralysis).* 1918.

Nathanson, Neal and Kew, Olen M. *From Emergence to Eradication: The Epidemiology of Poliomyelitis Deconstructed.* 2010.

Nixon, M.D., J.A. *Drinker's "Iron Lung" and Other Artificial Respirators.* 1938.

Noguchi, M.D., Hideyo and Kudo, M.D., Rokusaburo. *The Relation of Mosquitoes and Flies to the Epidemiology of Poliomyelitis.* 1917.

Oshinsky, David. *Polio: An American Story.* 2006.

Paul, John R. *A History of Poliomyelitis.* 1971.

———. *A Note on the Early History of Infantile Paralysis in the United States.* 1936.

Peabody, M.D., Francis W., Draper, M.D., George, and Dochez, M.D., A.R. *A Clinical Study of Acute Poliomyelitis: The Rockefeller Institute for Medical Research.* 1912.

Ratner, M.D., Herbert. *The Present Status of Polio Vaccines.* 1960.

Renne, Elisha P. *The 1917 Polio Outbreak in Montpelier, Vermont.* 2011.

Rissler, John. *Zur Kenntniss der Veränderungen des Nervensystems bei Poliomyelitis anterior acuta.* 1888.

Roberts, Kenneth and Galdone, Paul. *It Must Be Your Tonsils.* 1936.

Rockefeller Institute for Medical Research. *Studies from the Rockefeller Institute for Medical Research.* 1918.

Rogers, Naomi. *Dirt and Disease: Polio Before FDR.* 1992.

Roosevelt, E. and Brough, James. *An Untold Story: The Roosevelts of Hyde Park.* 1973.

Rosenow, E.C., Towne, E.B. and Hess, C.L. *The Elective Localization of Streptocci from Epidemic Poliomyelitis.* 1918.

Ross, M.D., LL.D., F.R.C.P., James and Bury, M.D., M.R.C.P., Judson S. *On Peripheral Neuritis: A Treatise.* 1893.

Ross, Jean C. *The First Polio Epidemic in the U.S., 1894.* 1992.

Ruhrah, M.D., John and Mayer, M.D., Erwin E. *Poliomyelitis In All Its Aspects.* 1917.

Russell, M.D., F.R.C.P., Ritchie W. *Paralytic Poliomyelitis: The Early Symptoms and the Effect of Physical Activity on the Course of the Disease.* 1949.

Sabin, M.D., Albert. *Experimental Poliomyelitis by the Tonsillopharyngeal Route with Special Reference to the Influence of Tonsillectomy on the Development of Bulbar Poliomyelitis.* 1938.

Salk, M.D., F.A.P.H.A., et. al. *Formaldehyde Treatment and Safety Testing of Experimental Poliomyelitis Vaccines.* 1954.

Sanderson, E. Dwight. *The Gypsy Moth in New Hampshire.* 1905.

Scheele, Charles-Williams. *The Chemical Essays of Charles-William Scheele.* 1901.

Scobey, M.D., Ralph. *Is Human Poliomyelitis Caused By An Exogenous Virus?* 1954.

Seguin, M.D., E.C. *Myelitis Following Acute Arsenical Poisoning (by Paris or Schweinfurth Green)*. 1882.

Spear, Robert J. *The Great Gypsy Moth War: A History of the First Campaign in Massachusetts to Eradicate the Gypsy Moth, 1890-1901.* 2005.

Talley, R.N., Charlotte. *TRACING THE SOURCES AND LIMITING THE SPREAD OF INFANTILE PARALYSIS*. 1916.

Taylor, M.D., Charles Fayette. *Infantile Paralysis and its Attendant Deformities*. 1867.

———. *Theory and Practice of the Movement Cure*. 1861.

Transactions of the Vermont State Medical Society for the Year 1894. 1895.

Trask, M.D., James D., et al. *Poliomyelitis Virus in Human Stools.* 1940.

Treadway, Walter L. *The Feeble-Minded Their Prevalence and Needs in The School of Arkansas*. 1916.

Underwood, M.D., Michael. *Treatise on the Diseases of Children in Two Parts*. 1789.

Vaughan, Dr.P.H., F.A.P.H.A. *Discussion of Poliomyelitis Papers.* 1936.

Whorton, James. *Before Silent Spring: Pesticides and Public Health in Pre-DDT America*. 1974.

Wickman I. Beiträge zur Kenntnis der Heine-Medinschen Krankheit (Poliomyelitis acuta und verwandter Erkrankungen). 1907.

———. *Acute Poliomyelitis Heine-Medin's Disease*. 1913.

Williams, Gareth. *Paralyzed with Fear: The Story of Polio*. 2013.

Williams, Marilyn Thornton. *Washing "The Great Unwashed" Public Baths in Urban America, 1840-1920*. 1991.

Wilson, John R. *Margin of Safety: The Story of the Poliomyelitis*

Vaccine. 1960.

Wyatt, H.V. *Before the Vaccines: Medical Treatments of Acute Paralysis in the 1916 New York Epidemic of Poliomyelitis*. 2014.

———. *The 1916 New York City Epidemic of Poliomyelitis: Where Did the Virus Come From?* 2011.

Notes

1. E. F. Hutchins, *Historical Summary, Poliomyelitis. International Committee for the Study of Infantile Paralysis* (Baltimore: Williams & Wilkins Co., 1932), p. 7.
2. Albert Sabin, Rocky Mountain Conference on Infantile Paralysis, *Problems in the Epidemiology of Poliomyelitis At Home and Among Our Armed Forces*, 1946.
3. Charles Badham, "Paralysis in Childhood: Four remarkable cases of suddenly induced paralysis in the extremities occurring in children without any apparent cerebral or cerebrospinal lesion," *London Medical Gazette* 17 (1834-35): 215.
4. Charles Fayette Taylor, M.D., *Infantile Paralysis and its Attendant Deformities* (Philadelphia: Lippincott, 1867) 6-7.
5. Ibid., 118.
6. "Hints to Mothers on the Treatment of their Children— From Teething to Teens," Eighteenth Edition (London: John Steedman & Co., undated).
7. Badham, 215.
8. Ibid., 216.
9. Michael Underwood, *Diseases of Children* (London: 1796) Vol. II, 53.
10. E. C. Seguin, M. D., "Myelitis Following Acute Arsenical Poisoning (By Paris Green or Schwein-Furth Green)," *Journal of Nervous and Mental Disease*, vol. IX, no. 4 (October 1882): 6.
11. Ibid., 9.
12. "Danger to Human Beings from Use of Paris Green," *Insect Life*, vol. 1, (1888): 142.
13. James Putnam and Edward Wyllys Taylor, "Is Acute Poliomyelitis Unusually Prevalent This Season?" *Boston Medical and Surgical Journal*, vol. CXXIX, no. 21, 1893, 509.
14. E. C. Seguin, M. D., "Myelitis Following Acute Arsenical Poisoning (By Paris Green or Schwein-Furth Green)," *Journal of Nervous and Mental Disease*, vol. IX, no. 4 (October 1882): 9.

15. Putnam and Taylor, 510.
16. James Ross, M.D. and Judson Bury, M.D., "On Peripheral Neuritis, A Treatise" (London: Charles Griffin and Company Limited, 1893) 331-333.
17. James Putnam, "On Motor Paralysis and Other Symptoms of Poisoning from Medicinal Doses of Arsenic," *Boston Medical and Surgical Journal*, vol. CXIX, no. 1 1888 : 1.
18. W.B. Hills, "Chronic Arsenic Poisoning," *Boston Medical & Surgical Journal*, vol.131 (1894): 453-478.
19. C. S. Caverly, "Preliminary Report of an Epidemic of Paralytic Disease, Occurring in Vermont, in the Summer of 1894," *Yale Medical Journal*, vol. I, no. 1, (1894): 4-7.
20. Ibid., p.4-7.
21. Anderson S. AYRESS, NP, "CUTANEOUS MANIFESTATIONS OF ARSENIC POISONING," *Archives of Dermatology and Syphilology* 30(1) (1934): 33–43.
22. Ibid., 26.
23. Transactions of the Vermont State Medical Society for the Year 1894. "History of an Epidemic of Acute Anterior Poliomyelitis," C. S. Caverly, 1895, 264-265.
24. O. W. Holmes, *Medical Essays* (Boston: 1899), 203, 253-253.
25. Caverly, "Preliminary Report of an Epidemic of Paralytic Disease," 33.
26. Ibid., 34.
27. Caverly, "Transactions of the Vermont State Medical Society," 260.
28. K. Landsteiner and E. Popper: Mikroskopische Präparate von einem menschlichen und zwei Affenrückenmarken. *Wien. klin. Wschr.*, 21: 1830, 1903.
29. O. Medin, "The Acute Stage of Infantile Paralysis," *The St. Paul Medical Journal* (1910): 215-216.
30. James Putnam, "Infectious Nervous Diseases," *The American Journal of the Medical Sciences*, vol. CIX (1895): 269.
31. Arthur Kallet and A. J. Schlink, *100,000,000 Guinea Pigs*, (Vanguard Press: 1933), 55-56.
32. W. H. Frost, "The Field Investigation of Epidemic Poliomyelitis (What The Health Officer Can Do Toward Solving A National Health Problem)," *Public Health Reports*, vol. XXV, no. 46, (1910), 1663.
33. Ibid., 1673.
34. Frost, 1673.
35. Charles Caverly, "Infantile Paralysis in Vermont," State Department of Public Health (1924), 53.
36. Kurt Schefczik and Klaus Buff, "The insecticide DDT decreases membrane potential and cell input resistance of cultured human liver cells," *Biochimica et Biophysica Acta (BBA) - Biomembranes*, vol. DCCLXXVI, Issue 2 (1984):

337-339.
37. Caverly, "Infantile Paralysis in Vermont," 28.
38. E. G. Packard, "Spray, O Spray," *Entomological News*, Volume 17, 1906, 256.
39. James Whorton, *Before Silent Spring* (Princeton University Press: 1974), 77.
40. W.C. O'Kane, C.H. Hadley, and W.A. Osgood, New Hampshire AES, Bulletin 183, 1917, 35.
41. Annual Report of the Department of Health, of the City of New York. (1916), Haven Emerson, 22.
42. Ibid., 24.
43. "Anna's Wail Made John a Prize Baby," *The New York Times*, 6 May 1916, 15.
44. Ibid., 15.
45. Ibid., 15.
46. "All Unite to Check Infant Paralysis," *The New York Times*, 30 June 1916, 8.
47. "MAYOR MOBILIZES CITY'S EMPLOYEES IN PARALYSIS WAR," *The New York Times*, 10 July 10 1916, 1.
48. "Children of the Slums," *The New York Times*, July 28, 1916.
49. "31 DIE OF PARALYSIS; 162 MORE ILL IN CITY," *The New York Times*, 15 July 1916, 16.
50. Ibid., 1.
51. Ibid., 1.
52. Ibid., 16.
53. "Crowded Public Baths," *The New York Times*, 9 July 1916.
54. "MAYOR MOBILIZES CITY'S EMPLOYEES IN PARALYSIS WAR," *The New York Times*, 10 July 1916, 1.
55. Ibid., 1.
56. Ibid., 1.
57. "A Monograph on the Epidemic of Poliomyelitis (Infantile Paralysis) in New York City in 1916," Department of Health, New York City, 1917.
58. "Rochester, N.Y., Tonsil-Adenoid Clinic and Hospital," Rochester Children's Clinic and Hospital, 1920, 455-457.
59. Ibid., 456-457.
60. Elliott Roosevelt & James Brough, *An Untold Story, The Roosevelts of Hyde Park* (New York: Dell Publishing, 1973), 159.
61. Kenneth Davis, *FDR: The Beckoning of Destiny* (New York: Putnam & Sons, 1971), 655.
62. *Rachel Lynn Palmer and Isadore M. Alpher, 40,000,000 Guinea Pig Children (New York: Vanguard Press, 1937), 141.*
63. *Science*, vol. 67, 1928, 357.
64. Talbert and Tayloe, Research Bulletin 183, 4.

65. Tom Harpole, "That Old-Time Profession," *Air & Space Magazine*, 7 March 2007.
66. Francis Weld Peabody, Alphonse Raymond Dochez, George Draper,"A Clinical Study of Acute Poliomyelitis," The Rockefeller Institute for Medical Research, New York, 1912, 71-72.
67. Philip Drinker and C. F. McKhann, "The Use Of A New Apparatus For The Prolonged Administration Of Artificial Respiration. A Fatal Case Of Poliomyelitis," *Journal of the American Medical Association* (1929): 1658–1660.
68. Eleanor Early, "Science's New Way To Save Life When Breathing Fails," *The Bismarck Tribune*, 2 January 1930.
69. "Man's First Call for Respirator Saves Him at Cost of Girl's Life," *Daily Capital Journal* (Salem, Oregon), 25 August 1930, 4.
70. Leonard C. Hawkins, *The Man in the Iron Lung*, Doubleday, 1956, 67.
71. "Health War Ordered On Paralysis: Dr. Parrish Authorized to Take Needed Steps to Halt Poliomyelitis Spread," *The Los Angeles Times*, 18 May 1934, 25.
72. "Infant Disease Shows Decline," *The Los Angeles Times*, 16 June 1934, 15.
73. Ibid., 15.
74. J. R. Paul, *A History of Poliomyelitis* (Yale University Press: 1971), 217.
75. Ibid., 218.
76. Ibid., 219-220.
77. Simon Flexner, "Epidemic (lethargic) encephalitis and allied conditions," *Journal of the American Medical Association*, (1923): 1688-93, 1785-89.
78. M. Brodie and W.H. Park, "Active immunization against Poliomyelitis, N.Y. St. J. Ned., 35: 1935; *Journal of the American Medical Association*, 105: 10: 9, 1935.
79. *Palmer, 141.*
80. Letter to Mrs. Franklin Roosevelt, Dec. 26, 1933. Rec. Off Sec. Ag.
81. Kallet, 52.
82. "Spraying an Island," *The New York Times*, 24 December 1944.
83. "DDT, the Army's Insect Powder, Strikes a Blow Against Typhus and for Pest Control," *The New York Times*, 4 July 1944.
84. Albert B. Sabin, "Paralytic Consequences of Poliomyelitis Infection in Different Parts of the World and in Different Population Groups," *American Journal of Public Health and the Nations Health* 41.10 (1951): 1215–1230.
85. Ibid., 1217.
86. J.K. Terres, *New Republic*, 114 (1946): 115.
87. *Public Health Reports* Vol. 63, No. 13 "Incidence of Poliomyelitis in 1947," 393.
88. "Mysterious 'Virus X' Strikes Los Angeles," *The News* (Frederick, Maryland), 22 December 1947, 1.

89. “Virus X Forces Hollywood Stars to Try Many Fancy Remedies,” *The Courier Journal* (Louisville, Kentucky) 2 March 1951, 24.
90. M. S. Biskind, "DDT Poisoning and the Elusive 'Virus X': A New Cause for Gastro-Enteritis," *American Journal of Digestive Diseases* 16: 79 (1949).
91. Ibid., 79.
92. “Insecticide is Denied Cause for Virus X,” *The Edwardsville Intelligencer* (Edwardsville, Illinois), 2 April 1949, 2.
93. “Starting a Campaign Against Polio in the Schools,” *The New York Times*, 7 June 1952, 40.
94. Ibid., 40.
95. William Bischoff, “Bigger Doses of DDT Needed,” *The Miami News*, 12 August 1952, 4.
96. “6 In Family Get Polio,” *The Corpus Christi Caller-Times* (Texas), 8 September 1952, 24.
97. *Morbidity and Mortality Weekly Report* Annual Supplement Vol. 9, No. 53, US Public Health Service.
98. Rachel Carson, *Silent Spring* (Houghton Mifflin Harcourt: 1962), 157.
99. Carson, 158.
100. “The Present State of Polio Vaccines,” *Illinois Medical Journal* (1960): 84.
101. Ibid., 84-85.
102. Ibid., 86-87.
103. Ibid., 88.
104. G. C. Brown, “Laboratory Data on the Detroit Poliomyelitis Epidemic 1958,” *Journal of the American Medical Association*, vol. CLXXII (February 20, 1960): 807–812.
105. G. R. Cameron and F. Burgess, “The Toxicity of D.D.T.,” *British Medical Journal* 1.4407 (1945): 865–871.

Printed in Great Britain
by Amazon

32862923R00162